# **THE BEST FOODS TO COOK SOUS VIDE**

*Simple Melt-in-Your-Mouth Recipes That Make Buying a Sous Vide Machine Worth It*

Fit and Sous

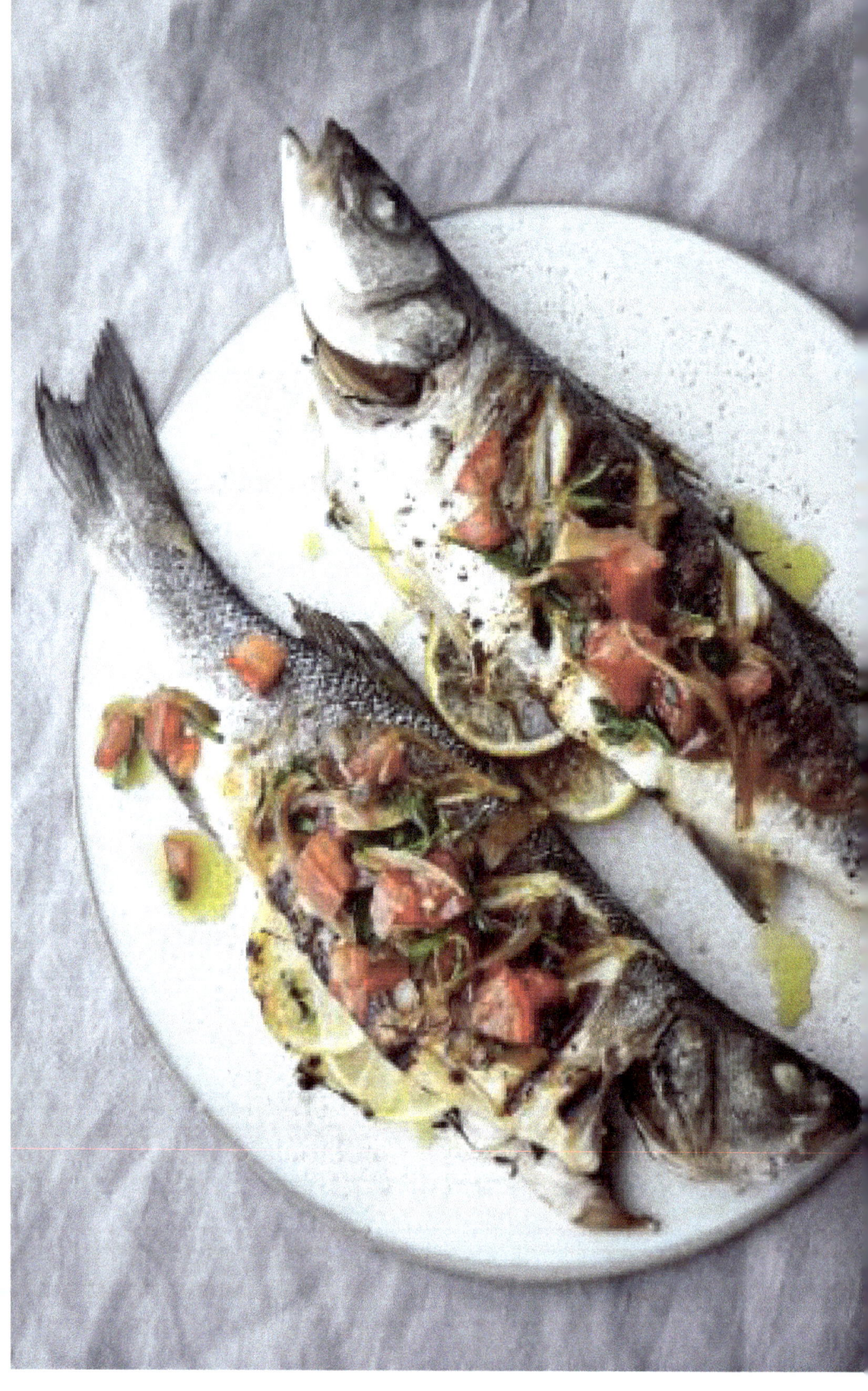

© Copyright 2020 by Fit and Sous- All rights reserved.

The following Book is reproduced below with the goal of providing information that is as accurate and reliable as possible. Regardless, purchasing this Book can be seen as consent to the fact that both the publisher and the author of this book are in no way experts on the topics discussed within and that any recommendations or suggestions that are made herein are for entertainment purposes only. Professionals should be consulted as needed prior to undertaking any of the action endorsed herein.

This declaration is deemed fair and valid by both the American Bar Association and the Committee of Publishers Association and is legally binding throughout the United States.

Furthermore, the transmission, duplication, or reproduction of any of the following work including specific information will be considered an illegal act irrespective of if it is done electronically or in print. This extends to creating a secondary or tertiary copy of the work or a recorded copy and is only allowed with the express written consent from the Publisher. All additional right reserved.

The information in the following pages is broadly considered a truthful and accurate account of facts, and as such, any inattention, use, or misuse of the information in question by the reader will render any resulting actions solely under their purview. There are no scenarios in which the publisher or the original author of this work can be in any fashion deemed liable for any hardship or damages that may befall them after undertaking information described herein.

Additionally, the information in the following pages is intended only for informational purposes and should thus be thought of as universal. As befitting its nature, it is presented without assurance regarding its prolonged validity or interim quality. Trademarks that are mentioned are done without written consent and can in no way be considered an endorsement from the trademark holder.

# Table of Contents

INTRODUCTION ..................................................................1

CHICKEN ..........................................................................8

    Easy Cheesy Chicken Balls......................................9

    Spice Turkey Dish ..................................................12

    Tempting Turkey in Orange Sauce........................13

    Italian Chicken Finger............................................16

    Flavorful Mustard Drumsticks ...............................18

    Cheesy Turkey Burgers .........................................20

    Delicious Thyme and Rosemary Turkey Legs.......22

    Pleasant Turkey Breast with Cloves ......................24

    Chicken Breast Meal .............................................27

    Delightful Spicy Adobo Chicken ...........................29

    Ginger Duck Breast ...............................................32

    Greek Meatballs....................................................35

Tasty Jamaican Jerk Chicken ................................................. 37

## MEAT ................................................................................ 39

Smokey Brisket ..................................................................... 41

Teriyaki Beef Ribs ................................................................. 43

Easy Lamb Chops ................................................................. 47

Tempting Lamb Chops and Mint Pistachio ........................... 49

Stuffed Beef Bell Peppers ..................................................... 52

Enticing Herb Crusted Lamb Rack ........................................ 54

Veal Chops ............................................................................ 58

Enjoyable Rosemary Meatballs with Yogurt ........................ 60

Ground Beef Kebab .............................................................. 63

Pleasant Teriyaki Skewered Lamb ........................................ 65

Lamb Chops & Mint Pistachio .............................................. 67

Flavorful Lamb Rack with Dijon Mustard ............................. 70

Quail Breast .......................................................................... 72

## PORK ................................................................................ 74

Pork with Tomatoes and Potatoes ........................................75

Ginger Pork ...........................................................................77

Easy Pork and Creamy Scallions Sauce ...............................78

Delicious Pork and Zucchini Ribbons ..................................79

Tasty Herbed Pork Loin ........................................................81

Enjoyable Red Pepper Salad and Pork Chops .....................83

Pleasant Fragrant Nonya Pork Belly ....................................85

Enjoyable Pork Chop with Corn ...........................................87

Mango Salsa and Pork ...........................................................89

Tempting Lemongrass Pork Chops ......................................91

Enticing Pork and Zucchini Ribbons ...................................93

Easy Herbed Pork Loin .........................................................95

## SIDE DISHES ......................................................................97

Tasty Trout with Pesto and Lemon Juice ............................98

Easy Garlic and Herbs Cod ...................................................99

Delicious Coconut Cream Sea Bass .................................. 100

Wild Salmon Steaks ............................................................ 102

Enticing Marinated Catfish Fillets ...................................... 104

Enjoyable Cilantro Trout ..................................................... 106

Shrimp Salad........................................................................ 108

Shrimp and Leek ................................................................. 110

Tasty Pumpkin Shrimp........................................................ 112

Enjoyable Miso Butter Cod................................................. 115

Yummy Dijon Cream Sauce with Salmon .......................... 117

Flavorful Mahi-Mahi Corn Salad......................................... 119

# INTRODUCTION

## The Sous Vide Cooking Method

A French word that means "under vacuum," sous vide is a technique of cooking under pressure. It is also called low-temperature long cooking, which means the process takes more time than with regular methods.

Sous vide refers to the process of vacuum-sealing food in a bag, then cooking it to a very precise temperature in a water bath. This technique produces results that are impossible to achieve through any other cooking method.

With traditional methods of cooking, you have less control over the temperature of the food itself. It can be overcooked on the outside, while only a small portion in the center achieves the temperature you want. This means that your food will lose flavor and end up with a dry, chewy texture.

There are three simple steps:

- Attach your precision cooker to a pot of water and set the time and temperature according to your desired level of doneness.
- Put your food in a sealable bag and clip it to the side of the pot.

- Finish by searing, grilling, or broiling the food to add a crispy, golden exterior layer

**The Sous Vide Cooking Method**

Food is placed into an airtight bag or a glass jar and put it in a water bath. Depending on the temperature you set, it can take up to 72 hours to achieve the desired results.

For red meat set your temperature to 55-60 °C or 130-140 F.

For poultry, set your temperature to 66-71 °C or 150-160 F.

Setting the correct temperature will ensure that your food is cooked perfectly and remains juicy and flavorful.

The Best Food to Cook Sous Vide:

- Tougher cuts of meat
- Eggs
- Pork
- Lamb
- Carrots
- Sausage
- Corn
- Biscuits
- Salmon
- Yogurt
- Crème Brulee
- French fries

The Worst Food to Cook Sous-Vide:

- Filleted fish
- Liver
- Filleted steaks
- Hollandaise

## Benefits of Using the Sous Vide Cooking Method

- The sous vide method of cooking ensures that your food is evenly cooked inside and out.
- It retains the juiciness and flavor of the food because the food is sealed in an airtight container or bag.
- Your food will come out in the same form you put into the bag or container, while with regular cooking methods, it may break into pieces.
- You'll have less pressure or stress about perfectly cooked and well-balanced meals. With sous vide will wipe away all your tensions by providing you tender, juicy, and well-cooked meal.
- Sous vide requires less attention than regular cooking methods, which require diligence to make sure it does not burn.
- When you use precise temperatures and time, you can expect very consistent results.
- The food is moist, juicy, and tender.
- Traditionally prepared food dries out and results in waste. For example, on average, traditionally cooked steak loses up to 40 percent of its volume due to drying out. Steak cooked via precision cooking loses none of its volume.

**Drawbacks of sous vide**

- You will need to the equipment
- Although this technique requires less energy and effort, it takes more time than other cooking methods.
- You can only cook one thing at a time because different foods require different temperature and time.
- Traditional cooking can require your constant attention; however, precision cooking with sous vide delivers consistently delicious and perfectly cooked food.

# CHICKEN

# Easy Cheesy Chicken Balls

**Servings:** 12

**Preparation Time:** 1 hour

**Per Serving:** Calories 352, Fat 5, Fiber 3, Carbs 7, Protein 5

**Ingredients:**

- 2 pounds ground chicken
- 4 tbsps onion, finely chopped
- 1/2 tsp garlic powder
- Salt and black pepper to taste
- 2 tbsps breadcrumbs
- 1 egg
- 64 small, diced cubes of mozzarella cheese
- 2 tbsps butter
- 6 tbsps panko
- 1 cup tomato sauce
- 1 oz grated Pecorino Romano cheese
- Chopped parsley

**Procedure:**

1. Firstly, prepare a water bath and place the Sous Vide in it.
2. Set to 146 F. In a bowl, mix the chicken, onion, salt, garlic powder, pepper and seasoned breadcrumbs.
3. Add the egg and combine well.
4. Then, form 32 medium-size balls and fill with a cube of cheese, make sure the mix covers the cheese well.
5. Place the balls in a vacuum-sealable bag and let chill for 20 minutes.
6. Then, release air by the water displacement method, seal and submerge the bag in the water bath. Cook for 45 minutes.
7. Once the timer has stopped, remove the balls. Heat the butter in a skillet over medium-high heat and add the panko.
8. Cook until toast.
9. As well cook the tomato sauce.
10. Now, in a servings dish, place the balls and glaze with the tomato sauce.
11. Top with the panko and cheese.
12. Finally, garnish with parsley.

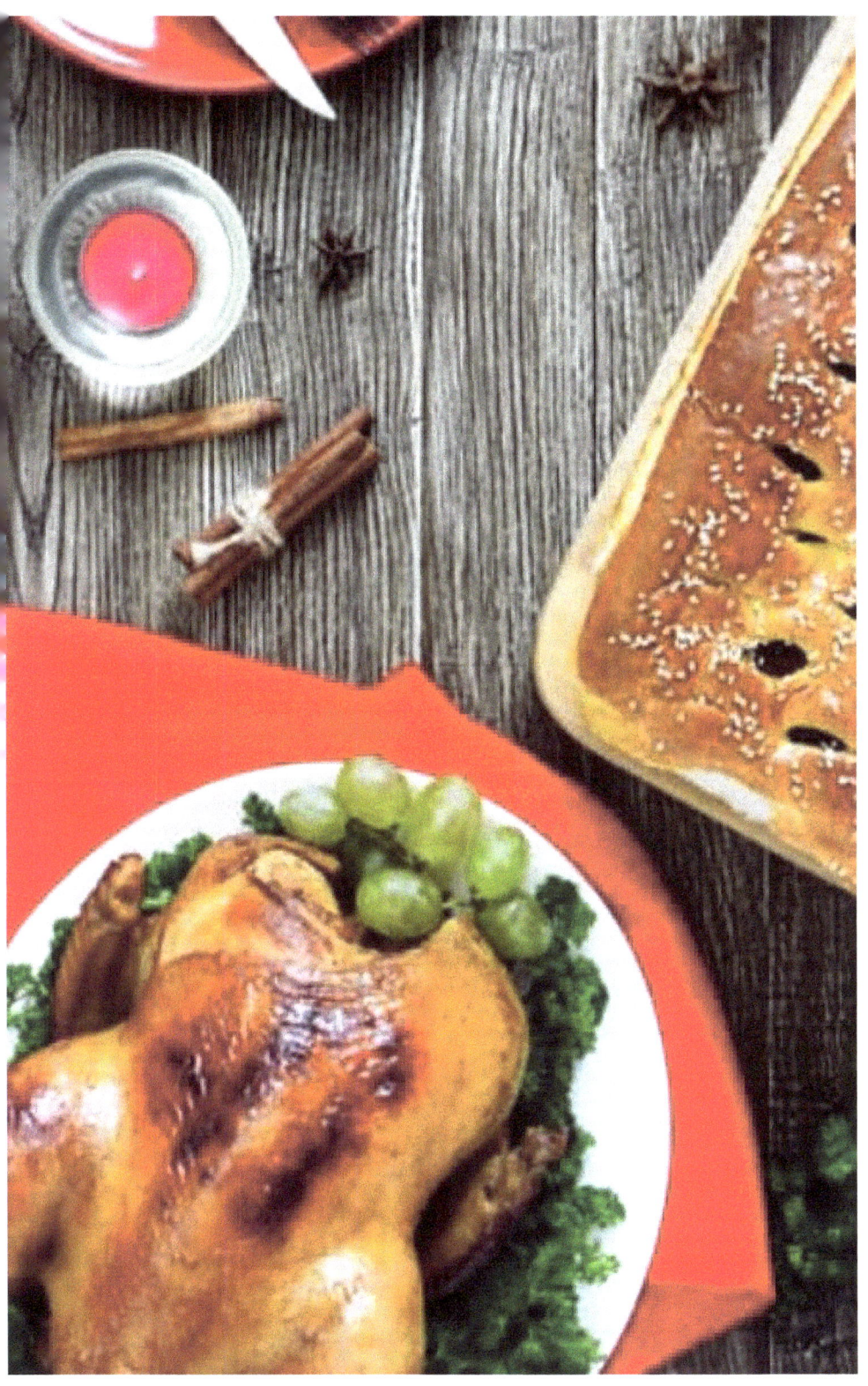

# Spice Turkey Dish

**Servings:** 8

**Preparation Time:** 1 hour

**Per Serving:** Calories 352, Fat 5, Fiber 3, Carbs 7, Protein 5

**Ingredients:**

- 2 turkey legs
- 2 tbsps olive oil
- 2 tbsps garlic salt
- 2 tsps black pepper
- 6 sprigs of thyme
- 2 tbsps rosemary

**Procedure:**

1. Firstly, prepare a water bath and place the Sous Vide in it.
2. Set to 146 F. Season the turkey with garlic, salt and pepper.
3. Place it in a vacuum-sealable bag.
4. Then, release air by the water displacement method, seal and submerge the bag in the bath.
5. Now, cook for 14 hours. Once done, remove the legs and pat it dry.

# Tempting Turkey in Orange Sauce

**Servings:** 4

**Preparation Time:** 1 hour 15 minutes

**Per Serving:** Calories 352, Fat 5, Fiber 3, Carbs 7, Protein 5

**Ingredients:**

- 2 pound turkey breasts, skinless and boneless
- 2 tbsps butter
- 6 tbsps fresh orange juice
- 1 cup chicken stock
- 2 tsps Cayenne pepper
- Salt and black pepper to taste

**Procedure:**

1. Firstly, rinse the turkey breasts under cold running water and pat dry. Set aside.
2. In a medium bowl, combine orange juice, chicken stock, Cayenne pepper, salt, and pepper.
3. Then, mix well and place the meat into this marinade. Refrigerate for 20 minutes.

4. Now, place the meat along with marinade into a large vacuum-sealable bag and cook en sous vide for 40 minutes at 122 F.
5. In a medium non-stick saucepan, melt the butter over a medium-high temperature.
6. Remove the meat from the bag and add it to the saucepan.
7. Finally, fry for 2 minutes and remove from the heat.

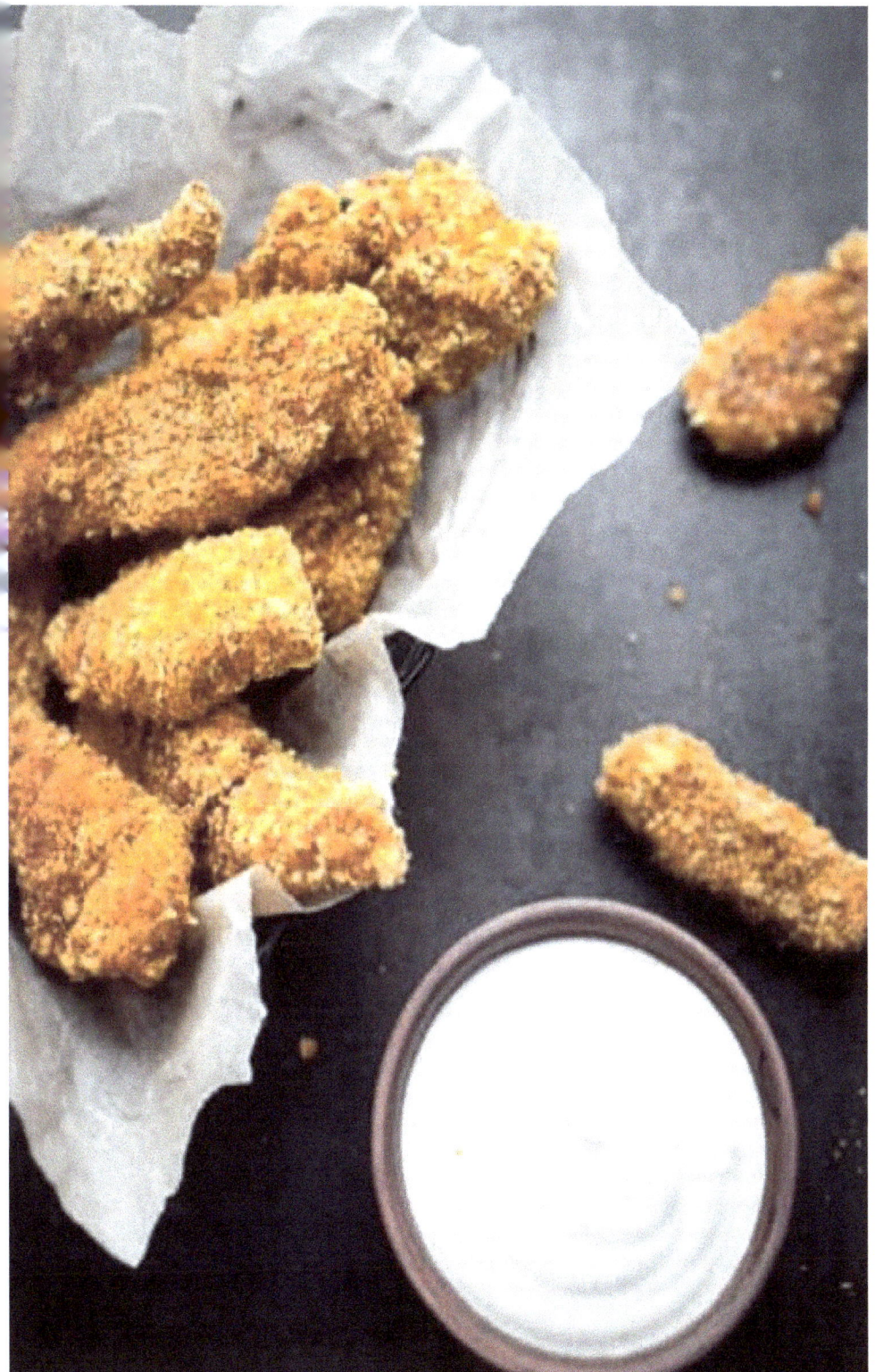

# Italian Chicken Finger

**Servings:** 6

**Preparation Time:** 2 hours

**Per Serving:** Calories: 424, Protein: 17.5g, Carbs: 17.5g, Fats: 33.3g

**Ingredients:**

- 2 lbs chicken breast, boneless skinless
- 2 cups almond flour
- 2 tsps minced garlic
- Salt and pepper to taste
- 1 tsp cayenne pepper
- 2 tbsps mixed Italian herbs
- 2 eggs, beaten
- 1/2 cup olive oil

**Procedure:**

1. Firstly, rinse the meat under cold running water and pat dry with a kitchen paper.
2. Season with mixed Italian herbs and place in a large Ziploc.

3. Seal the bag and cook en sous vide for 2 hours at 157 degrees F.
4. Remove from the water bath and set aside.
5. Now, combine together flour, salt, cayenne, Italian herbs, and pepper in a bowl and set aside.
6. In a separate bowl, beat the eggs and set them aside.
7. Heat olive oil in a large skillet over medium-high heat.
8. Dip the chicken into the beaten egg and coat with the flour mixture.
9. Finally, fry for 5 minutes on each side or until golden brown.

# Flavorful Mustard Drumsticks

**Servings:** 10

**Preparation Time:** 2 hours 50 minutes

**Per Serving:** Calories: 658, Protein: 53.5g, Carbs: 0.8g, Fats: 53.5g

**Ingredients:**

- 4 pounds chicken drumsticks
- 1/2 cup Dijon mustard
- 4 garlic cloves, crushed
- 4 tbsps coconut aminos
- 2 tsps pink Himalayan salt
- ½ tsp ground black pepper

**Procedure:**

1. Firstly, rinse drumsticks under cold running water.
2. Drain in a large colander and set aside.
3. Then, in a small bowl, combine Dijon mustard with crushed garlic, coconut aminos, salt, and pepper.
4. Now, spread the mixture over the meat with a kitchen brush and place in a large Ziploc bag.
5. Finally, seal the bag and cook en sous vide for 2 hours and 45 minutes at 157 degrees F.

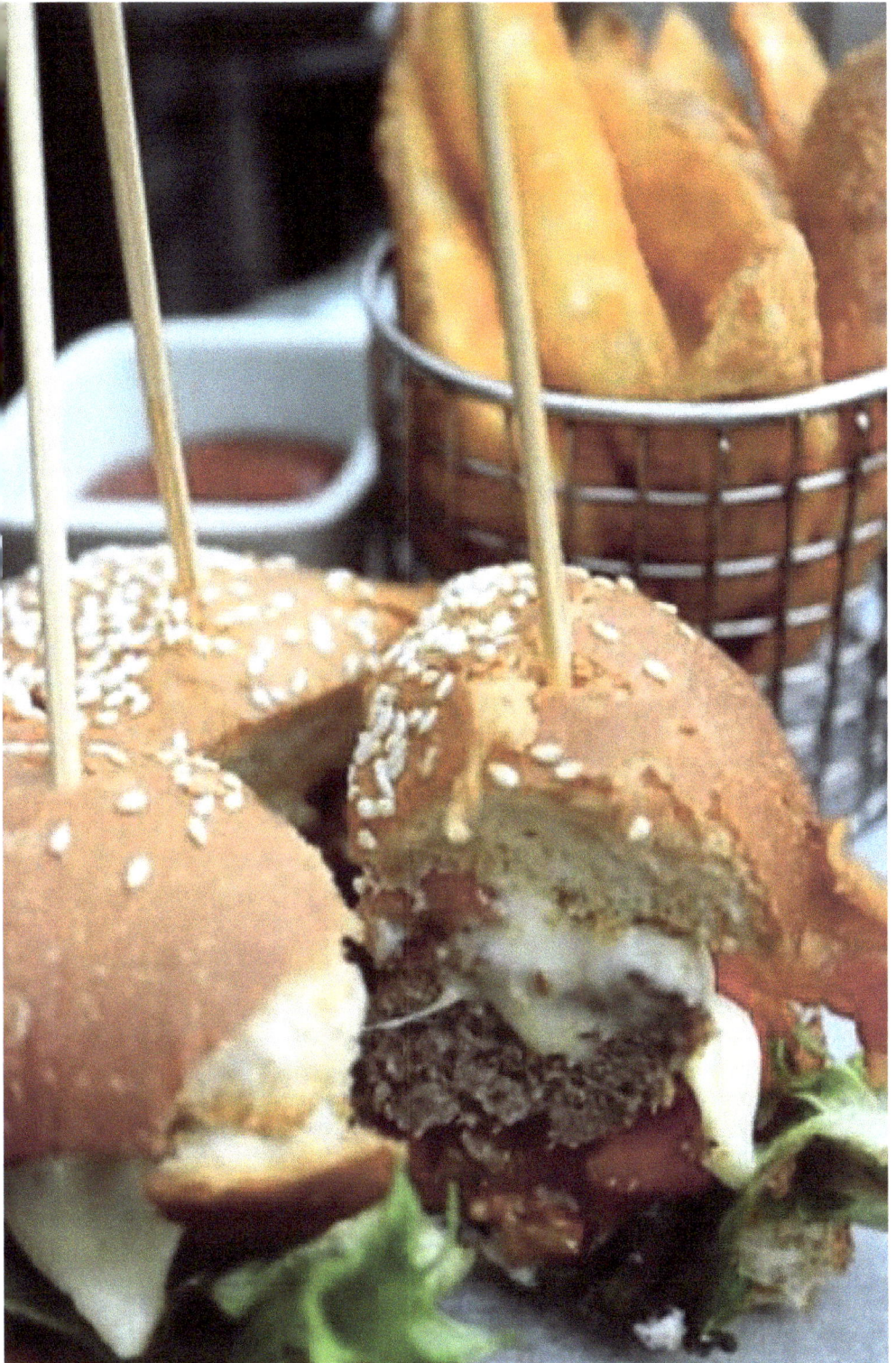

# Cheesy Turkey Burgers

**Servings:** 6

**Preparation Time:** 2 hours

**Per Serving:** Calories 352, Fat 5, Fiber 3, Carbs 7, Protein 5

**Ingredients:**

- 6 tsps olive oil
- 1½ pounds ground turkey
- 16 cream crackers, crushed
- 2½ tbsps chopped fresh parsley
- 2 tbsps chopped fresh basil
- ½ tbsp Worcestershire sauce
- ½ tbsp soy sauce
- ½ tsp garlic powder
- 1 egg
- 6 buns, toasted
- 6 tomato slices
- 6 Romaine lettuce leaves
- 6 slices Monterey Jack cheese

**Procedure:**

1. Prepare a water bath and place the Sous Vide in it. Set to 148 F.
2. Combine the turkey, crackers, parsley, basil, soy sauce and garlic powder. Add the egg and mix using your hands.
3. In a baking sheet with wax pepper, with the mixture, create 6 patties and place them.
4. Cover it and transfer into the fridge
5. Remove the patties from the fridge and place it in three vacuum-sealable bags. Release air by the water displacement method, seal and submerge the bag in the water bath. Cook for 1 hour and 15 minutes.
6. Once the timer has stopped, remove the patties.
7. Discard the cooking juices.
8. Heat the olive oil in a skillet over high heat and place the patties. Sear for 45 seconds per side.
9. Place the patties over the toasted buns.
10. Top with tomato, lettuce and cheese. Serve.

# Delicious Thyme and Rosemary Turkey Legs

**Servings:** 8

**Preparation Time:** 8 hours

**Per Serving:** Calories 352, Fat 5, Fiber 3, Carbs 7, Protein 5

**Ingredients:**

- 10 tsps butter, melted
- 20 garlic cloves, minced
- 4 tbsps dried rosemary
- 2 tbsps cumin
- 2 tbsps thyme
- 4 turkey legs

**Procedure:**

1. First, prepare a water bath and place the Sous Vide in it. Set to 134 F.
2. Combine the garlic, rosemary, cumin, thyme and butter. Rub the turkey with the mixture.
3. Then, place the turkey in a vacuum-sealable bag.
4. Release air by the water displacement method, seal and submerge the bag in the water bath. Cook for 8 hours

5. Once the timer has stopped, remove the turkey.
6. Reserve the cooking juices.
7. Heat the grill over high heat and put the turkey.
8. Sprinkle the cooking juices.
9. Now, turn around and sprinkle more juices.
10. Set aside and allow to cool.
11. Finally, serve.

# Pleasant Turkey Breast with Cloves

**Servings:** 12

**Preparation Time:** 2 hours

**Per Serving:** Calories 352, Fat 5, Fiber 3, Carbs 7, Protein 5

**Ingredients:**

- 4 pounds turkey breast, sliced
- 4 garlic cloves, minced
- 1 cup olive oil
- 4 tbsps Dijon mustard
- 4 tbsps lemon juice
- 2 tsps fresh rosemary, finely chopped
- 2 tsps cloves, minced
- Salt and black pepper to taste

**Procedure:**

1. Firstly, in a large bowl, combine olive oil with mustard, lemon juice, garlic, rosemary, cloves, salt, and pepper.
2. Mix until well incorporated and add turkey slices. Soak and refrigerate for 30 minutes before cooking.

3. Then, remove from the refrigerator and transfer to 2 vacuum-sealable bags.
4. Now, seal the bags and cook en Sous Vide for one hour at 149 F.
5. Finally, remove from the water bath and serve.

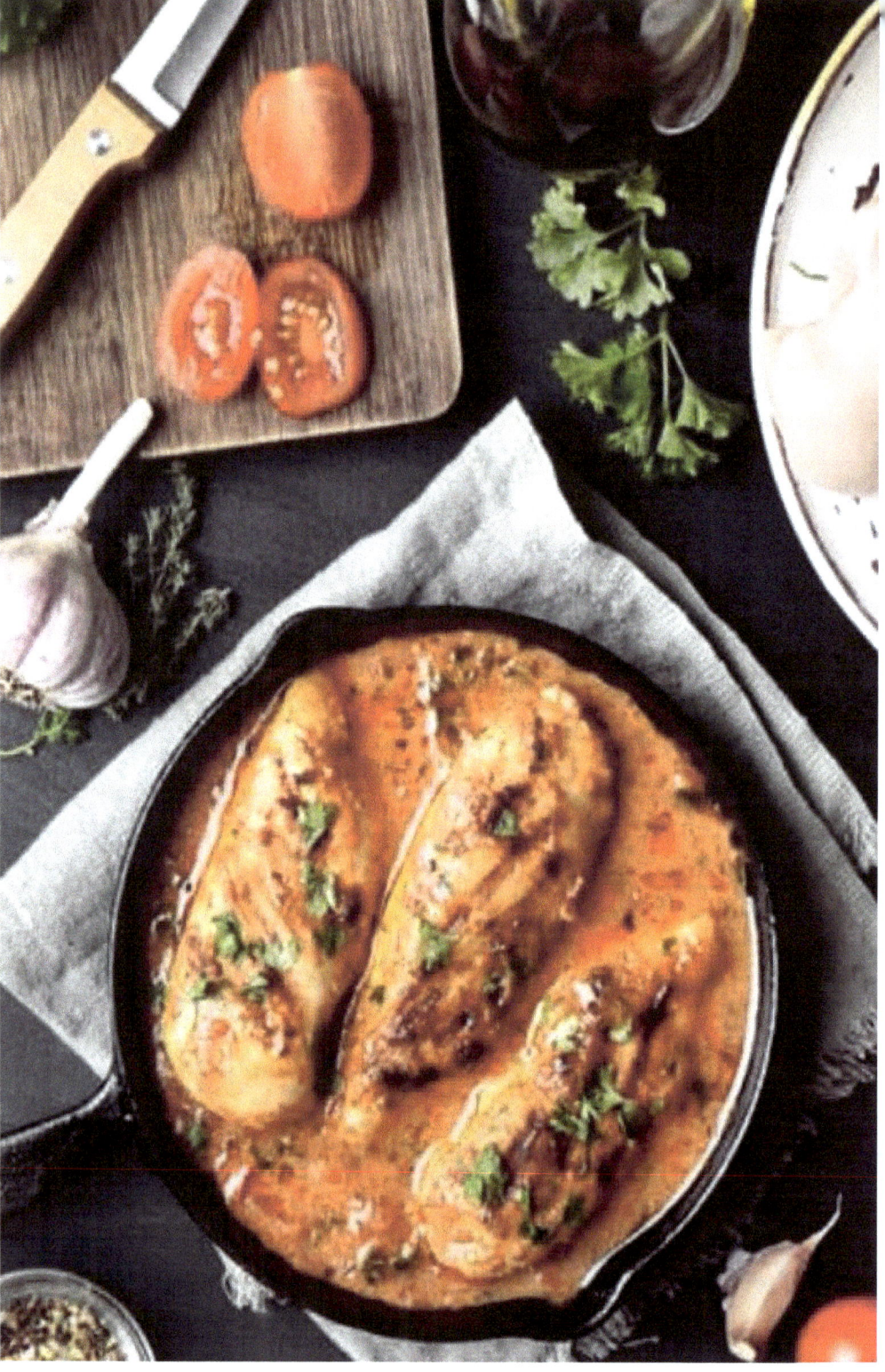

# Chicken Breast Meal

**Servings:** 4

**Preparation Time:** 1 hour

**Per Serving:** Calories: 150 Carbohydrate: 0g Protein: 18g Fat: 8g Sugar: 0g Sodium: 257mg

**Ingredients:**

- 2-pieces boneless chicken breast
- Salt and pepper as needed
- Garlic powder as needed

**Procedure:**

1. First, prepare your water bath using your Sous Vide immersion circulator, and increase the temperature to 150-degrees Fahrenheit
2. Then, carefully drain the chicken breast and pat dry using a kitchen towel
3. Season the breast with garlic powder, pepper and salt
4. Now, place in a resealable bag and seal using the immersion method
5. Submerge and cook for 1 hour
6. Finally, serve!

**Special Tips**

Remember that the time it takes to Sous Vide chicken breast depends on their size. If the breast is 1 inch in length, it will take 1 hour and if it is 2 inches long, it will take 2 hours, and so on....

# Delightful Spicy Adobo Chicken

**Servings:** 4

**Preparation Time:** 2 hours

**Per Serving:** Calories: 320 Carbohydrate: 33g Protein: 16g Fat: 14g Sugar: 3g Sodium: 255mg

**Ingredients:**

- 4 chicken leg quarters
- 4 garlic cloves, crushed
- 1/2 teaspoon whole black peppercorns
- 1 tablespoon molasses
- 1/2 cup dark soy sauce
- Salt as needed
- 1 tablespoon canola oil
- 1 Worcestershire sauce
- 2 bay leaves
- 1/2 cup white vinegar

**Procedure:**

1. First, mix the soy sauce, Worcestershire, peppercorns, molasses, garlic, bay leaf and salt.

2. Then, add the chicken legs in a Sous Vide bag with the marinade and refrigerate for 12 hours or overnight.
3. Prepare your Sous Vide water bath, using your immersion circulator, and raise the temperature to 165-degrees Fahrenheit
4. Submerge the chicken and cook for 2 hours
5. Remove the chicken legs from the bag and air dry for 10-15 minutes.
6. Sear over medium heat in a non-stick pan with canola oil
7. Now, add the sauce from the bag to the pan and keep cooking until you have reached the desired consistency
8. Finally, serve the chicken with sauce!

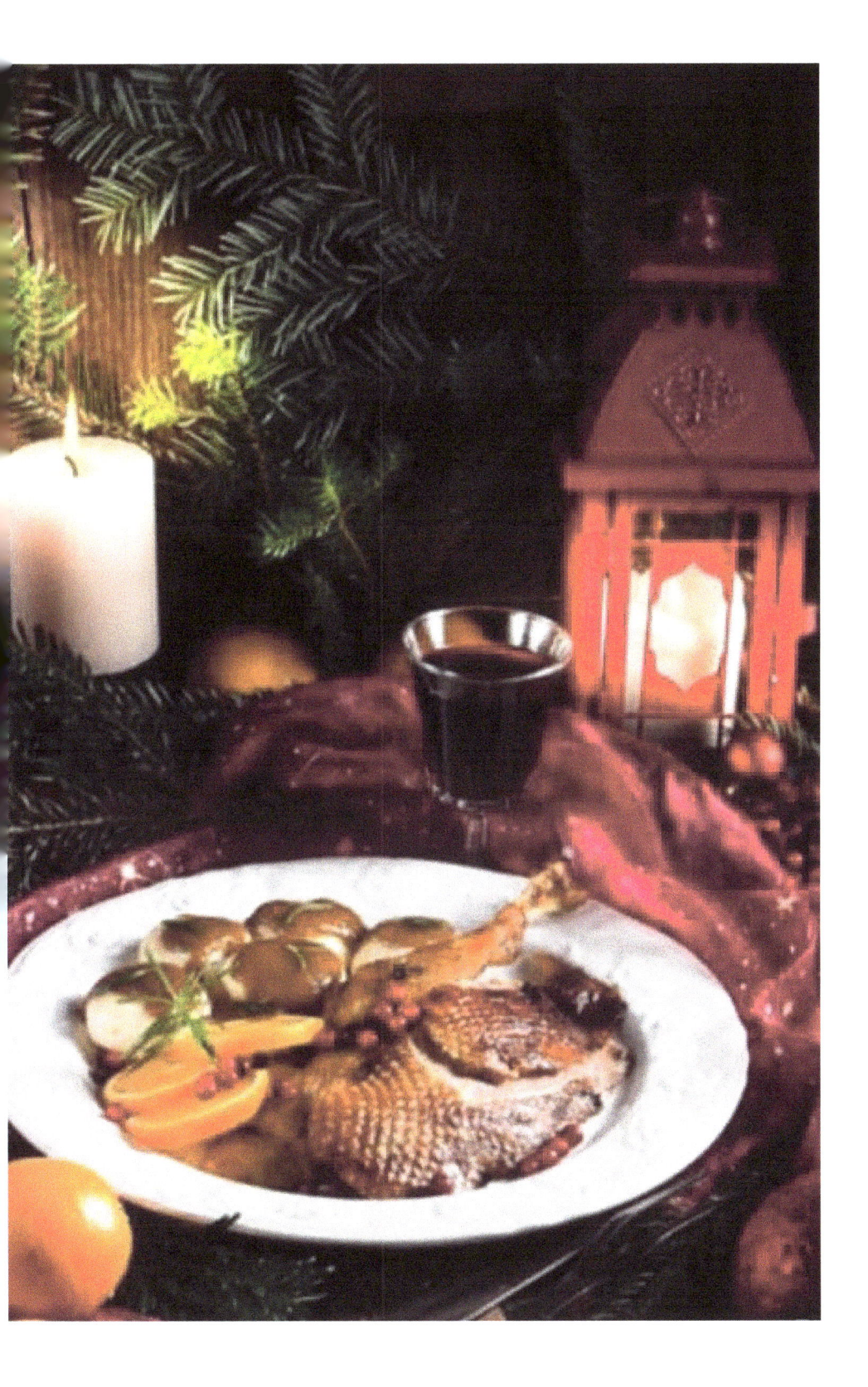

# Ginger Duck Breast

**Servings:** 4

**Preparation Time:** 2 hours

**Per Serving:** Calories: 365 Carbohydrate: 19g Protein: 18g Fat: 25g Sugar: 13g Sodium: 63mg

**Ingredients:**

- 4 boneless duck breasts
- Kosher salt and pepper as needed
- 2-inches fresh ginger, peeled and sliced thinly
- 4 garlic cloves, thinly sliced
- 3 teaspoons sesame oil

**Procedure:**

1. First, prepare your water bath using your Sous Vide immersion circulator, and raise the temperature to 135-degrees Fahrenheit
2. Season the duck breasts with pepper and salt
3. Then, put the breasts in a zip bag and add the ginger, sesame oil and garlic
4. Seal using the immersion method, and cook for 2 hours

5. Remove the duck and discard the garlic, ginger and cooking liquid
6. Place the duck breast in a cold, non-stick skillet and put it over a high heat
7. Cook the breast with the skin side down for about 30 seconds, flip, and cook for another 30 seconds
8. Now, place the breasts on a cutting board to rest for 5 minutes
9. Finally, slice the breasts and serve with your desired side dishes

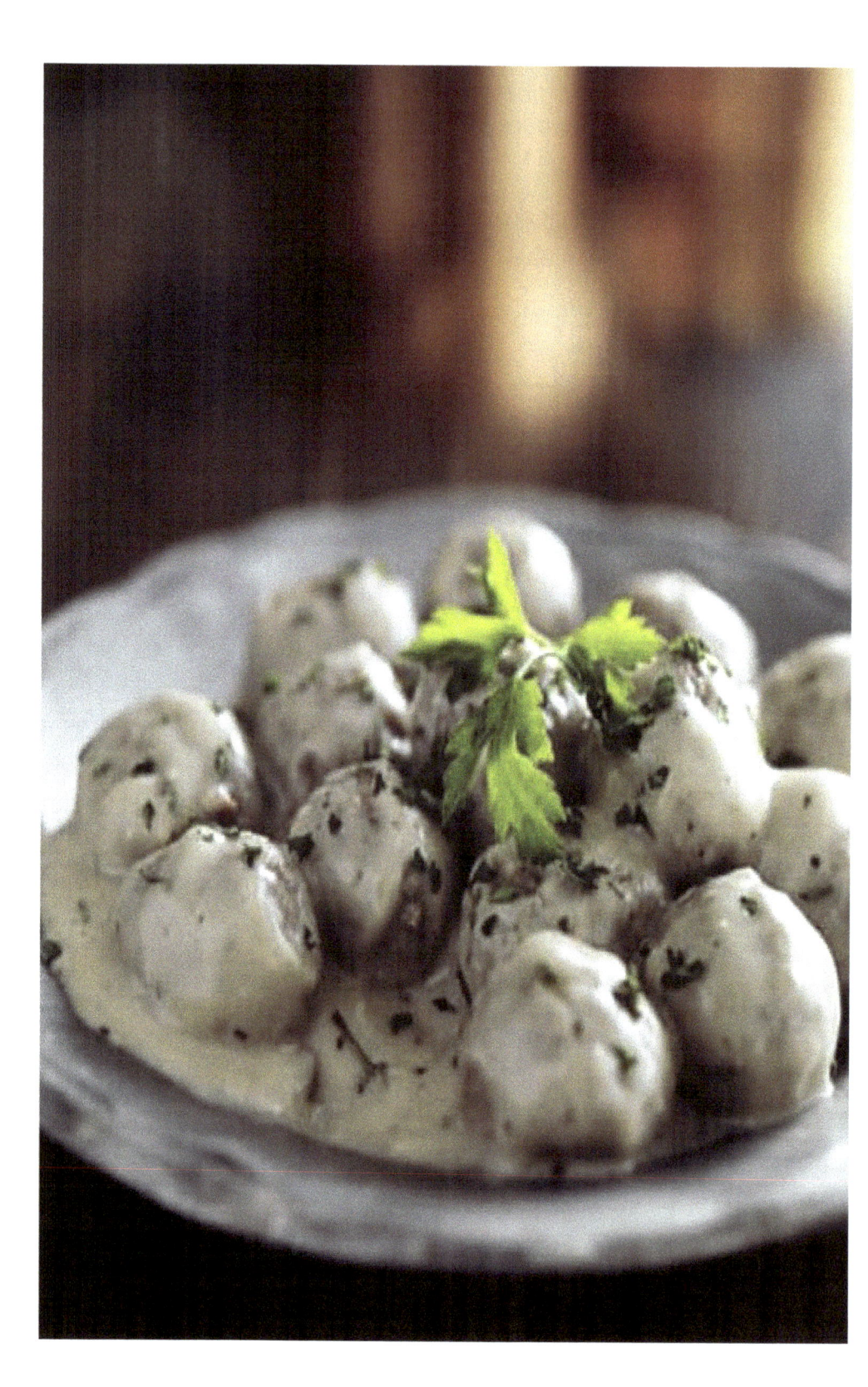

# Greek Meatballs

**Servings:** 8

**Preparation Time:** 2 hours 20 minutes

**Per Serving:** Calories: 238 Carbohydrate: 3g Protein: 8g Fat: 21g Sugar: 2g Sodium: 332mg

**Ingredients:**

- 2 lbs ground chicken
- 2 tablespoons extra-virgin olive oil
- 4 garlic cloves, minced
- 2 teaspoons fresh oregano, minced
- 2 teaspoons kosher salt
- 1 teaspoon grated lemon zest
- 1 teaspoon freshly ground black pepper
- 1/2 cup panko bread crumbs
- Lemon wedges for serving

**Procedure:**

1. First, prepare your Sous Vide water bath, using your immersion circulator, and raise the temperature to 146-degrees Fahrenheit

2. Add the garlic, olive oil, chicken, oregano, lemon zest, salt, and pepper in a medium-sized bowl
3. Mix well everything using your hands and gently mix in the panko bread crumbs
4. Form the mixture into 14 balls
5. Then, put the balls in a resealable bag and seal using the immersion method
6. Submerge the bag and cook for 2 hours
7. Remove the bag and transfer the balls to a baking sheet (lined with foil)
8. Set your broiler to high heat
9. Now, broil the balls for 5-7 minutes until they turn brown
10. Finally, serve with lemon wedges

# Tasty Jamaican Jerk Chicken

**Servings:** 6

**Preparation Time:** 3 hours

**Per Serving:** Calories: 330 Carbohydrate: 4g Protein: 24g Fat: 23g Sugar: 1g Sodium: 311mg

**Ingredients:**

- 4 lbs chicken wings
- 4 tablespoons jerk seasoning
- 1/2 cup fresh cilantro for garnishing, chopped

**Procedure:**

1. Firstly, prepare your Sous Vide water bath using your immersion circulator, and increase the temperature to 145-degrees Fahrenheit
2. Put the chicken and jerk seasoning in a resealable, heavy-duty plastic bag and seal the bag using the immersion method
3. Then, carefully transfer the bag under the preheated water bath and allow to cook for about 3 hours

4. Once done, take the bag out from the water and remove the wings, pat the wings dry with kitchen towel
5. Heat up your grill to high, and put the wings under it
6. Now, lower down the heat of your grill to medium and cook the chicken until crispy and slightly brown
7. Remove from the grill and add some jerk paste
8. Garnish with chopped cilantro
9. Finally, serve

# MEAT

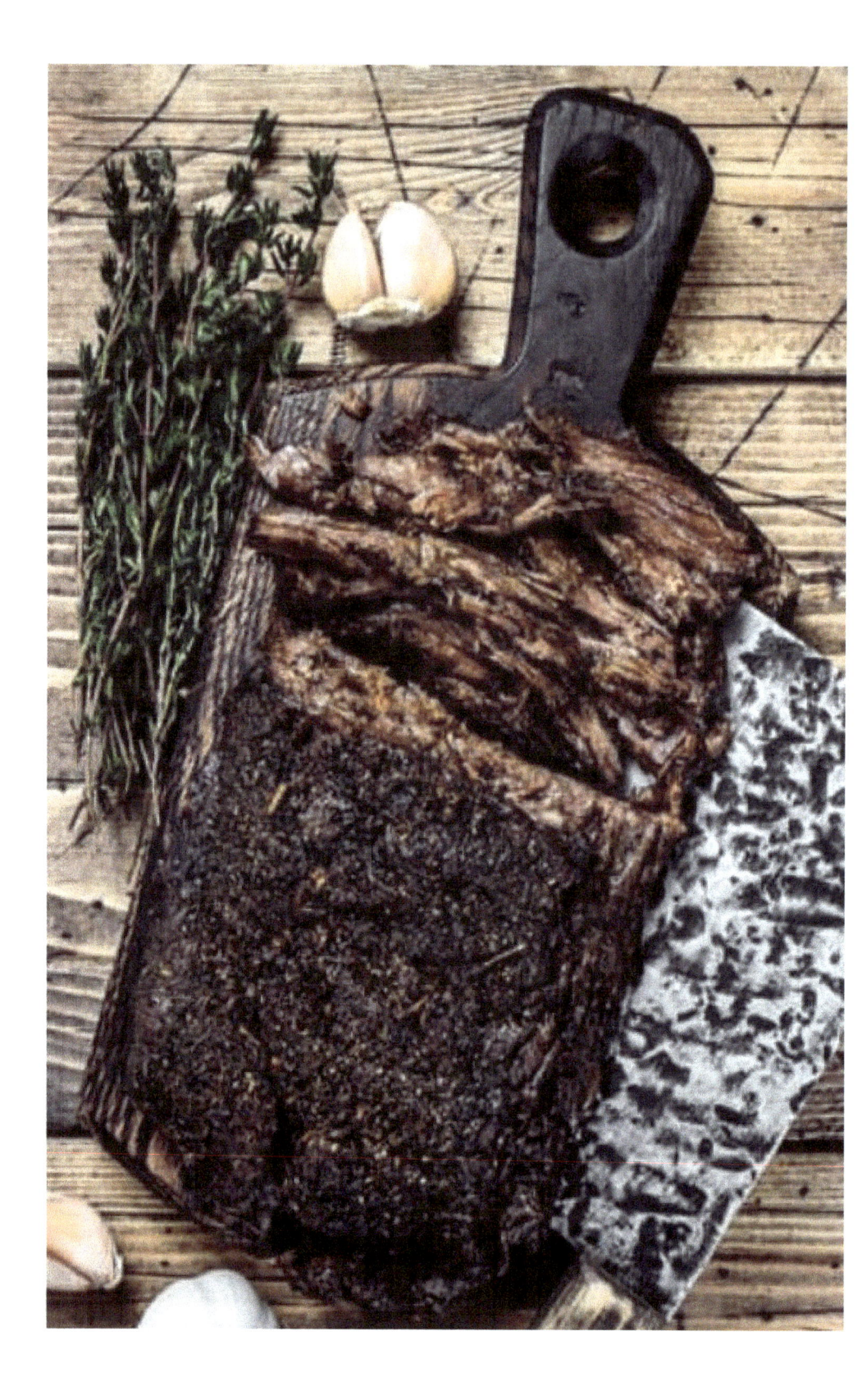

# Smokey Brisket

**Servings:** 8

**Preparation Time:** 24 hours

**Per Serving:** Calories 352, Fat 5, Fiber 3, Carbs 7, Protein 5

**Ingredients:**

- 5 pounds grass-fed beef brisket
- 1 tablespoon salt
- 4 teaspoons ground black pepper

**Procedure:**

1. First, attach the sous vide immersion circulator to a Cambro container or pot with water using an adjustable clamp and preheat water to 135°F.
2. Season brisket with salt and black pepper generously.
3. Place brisket in a cooking pouch.
4. Seal pouch tightly after removing the excess air.
5. Then, place pouch in sous vide bath and set the cooking time for 24 hours.
6. Cover the sous vide bath with plastic wrap to minimize water evaporation.

7. Add water intermittently to keep the water level up.
8. Remove pouch from the sous vide bath and open carefully.
9. Remove brisket from pouch and pat dry completely with paper towels.
10. Season brisket once again with salt and black pepper.
11. Heat a cast-iron skillet over medium-high heat and sear brisket for 2-3 minutes on each side.
12. Now, remove from heat and transfer to a cutting board for 5-10 minutes.
13. Finally, cut into desired slices and serve.

# Teriyaki Beef Ribs

**Servings: 8**

**Preparation Time:** 72 hours

**Per Serving:** Calories 352, Fat 5, Fiber 3, Carbs 7, Protein 5

**Ingredients:**

For Ribs:

- 8 pounds beef ribs, cut into three portions
- 1 cup sugar
- 1 cup salt
- Vegetable oil, as required

For Teriyaki Glaze:

- 2 cups mirin
- 1 cup sake
- 1 cup dark soy sauce

For Chili Oil:

- 6 tablespoons vegetable oil
- 8 tablespoons garlic, chopped

- 8 tablespoons fresh ginger, grated
- 2 green chilis, finely chopped

**Procedure:**

1. First, in a large bowl of water, dissolve sugar and salt.
2. Add beef ribs and set aside for 1-2 hours.
3. Remove ribs from brine and pat dry with paper towels.
4. Attach the sous vide immersion circulator to a Cambro container or pot with water using an adjustable clamp and preheat water to 132°F.
5. Divide ribs into two large cooking pouches.
6. Seal pouches tightly after removing the excess air.
7. Then, place pouches in sous vide bath and set the cooking time for 72 hours.
8. Cover the sous vide bath with plastic wrap to minimize water evaporation.
9. Add water intermittently to keep the water level up.
10. For teriyaki glaze: while ribs cook, add mirin, sake, and soy sauce to a pan and bring to a boil.
11. Now, reduce heat and simmer for 10 minutes, stirring occasionally.
12. For chili oil: in another pan, add oil, garlic, ginger, and green chili over low heat and cook until fragrant.

13. Finally, remove pouches from the sous vide bath and open carefully.
14. Remove ribs from pouch and pat dry with paper towels.
15. In a cast-iron skillet, heat oil over medium-high heat and sear ribs for 1 minute on each side.
16. Place ribs on a servings platter and top with glaze and chili oil. Serve immediately.

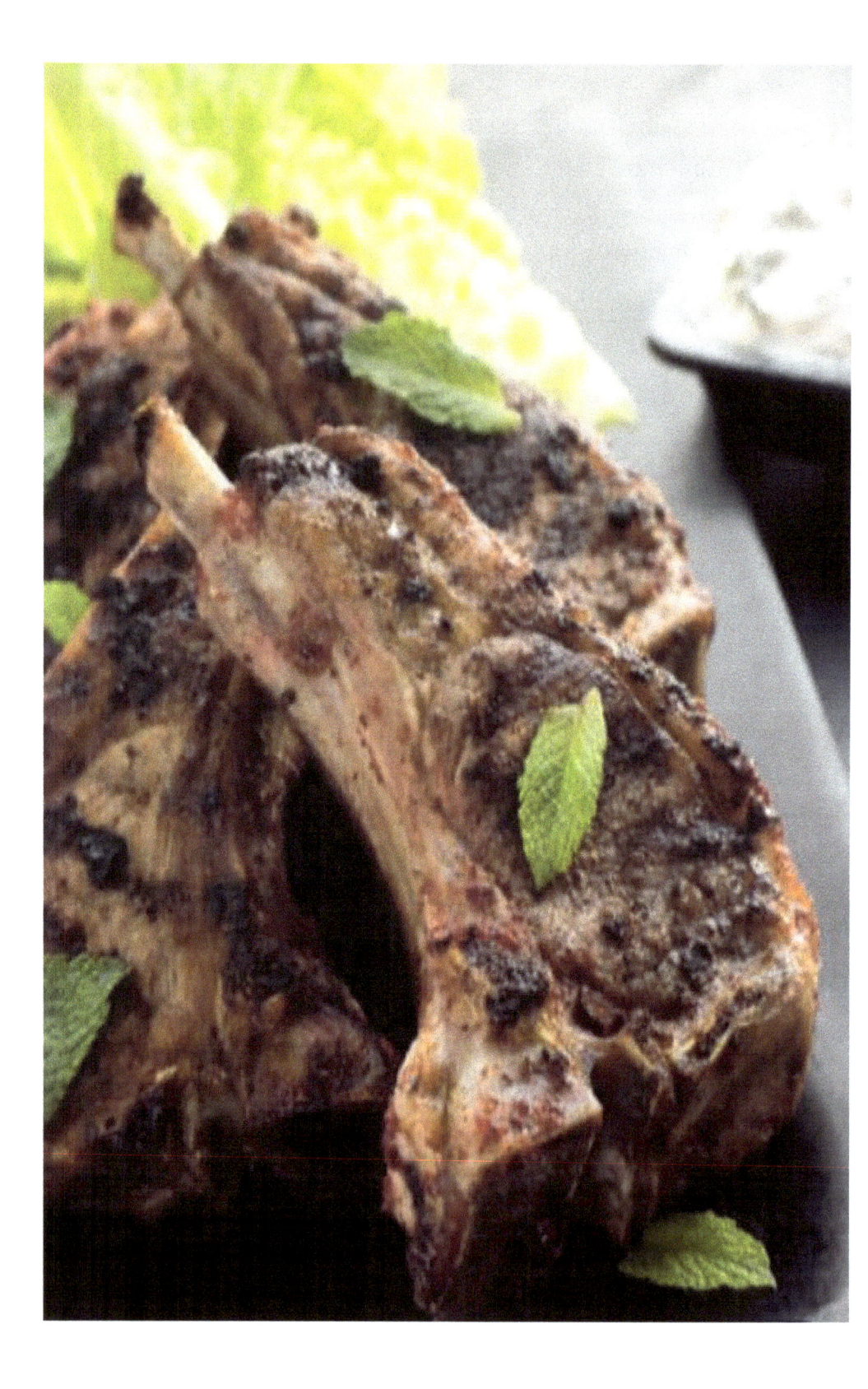

# Easy Lamb Chops

**Servings:** 4

**Preparation Time:** 2 hours

**Per Serving:** Calories 334, Fat 33, Fiber 3, Carbs 14, Protein 7

**Ingredients:**

- 4 lamb loin chops
- Salt and pepper as needed
- 3 teaspoons spice blend
- 8 prunes
- 2 tablespoons honey
- 2 teaspoons extra-virgin olive oil

**Procedure:**

1. Firstly, prepare the Sous Vide water bath using your immersion circulator and increase the temperature to 134-degrees Fahrenheit
2. Take the lamb chops and season them thoroughly with salt and pepper. Rub the lamb chops with the spice blend

3. Then, pace the chops in a zip bag, add the prunes and honey, and seal using the immersion method
4. Submerge it underwater and cook for 2 hours
5. Once done, remove the lamb chops and save prunes and cooking liquid
6. Take out the cooked lamb chops and pat them dry using a kitchen towel
7. Place an iron skillet over medium heat for about 5 minutes
8. Add the olive oil and the lamb chops and sear for 30 seconds per side
9. Now, put on a servings plate and let it stay for 5 minutes
10. Finally, drizzle some of the cooking liquid from the bag over the chops and serve with the prunes

# Tempting Lamb Chops and Mint Pistachio

**Servings:** 8

**Preparation Time:** 2 hours

**Per Serving:** Calories 334, Fat 33, Fiber 3, Carbs 14, Protein 7

**Ingredients:**

- 4 full racks lamb sliced into chops
- Kosher salt and black pepper as needed
- 2 cups packed fresh mint leaves
- 1 cup unsalted pistachio nuts, shelled
- 1 cup packed fresh parsley
- 1 cup scallion, sliced
- 6 tablespoons lemon juice
- 4 cloves garlic, minced
- 12 tablespoons extra-virgin olive oil

**Procedure:**

1. Firstly, prepare the Sous Vide water bath using your immersion circulator and raise the temperature to 125-degrees Fahrenheit
2. Season the lamb with salt and pepper

3. Put in a zip bag and seal using the immersion method. Cook for 2 hours
4. After 20 minutes, take the lamb out and set the grill to high
5. Then, add the mint, parsley, pistachios, scallions, garlic, and lemon juice in a food processor and form a paste
6. Drizzle 4 tablespoons of olive oil as you process, and keep going until you have a smooth paste
7. Season with salt and pepper
8. Now, brush your cooked lamb with 2 tablespoons of olive oil and grill for 1 minute per side
9. Finally, serve the chops with pesto

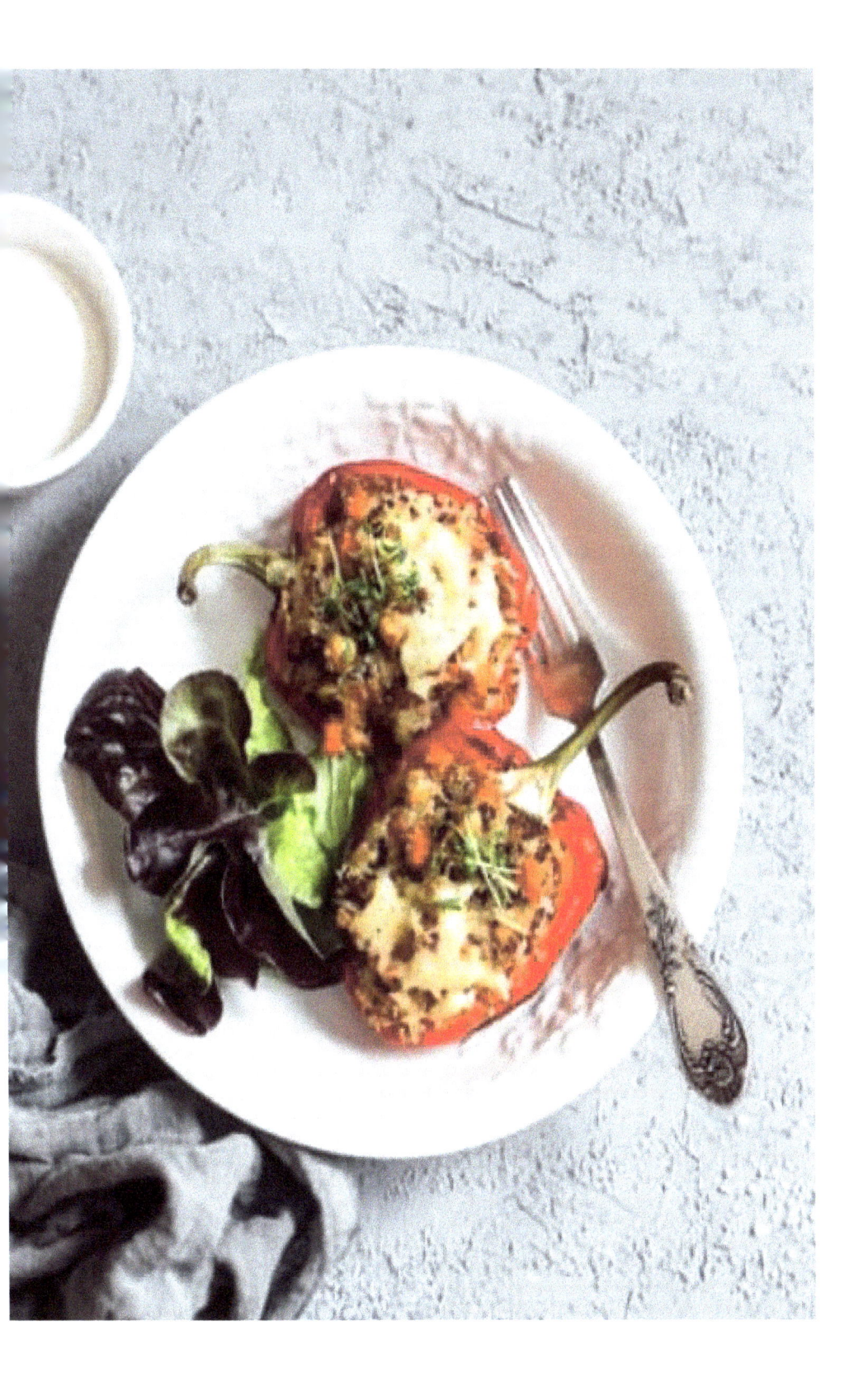

# Stuffed Beef Bell Peppers

**Servings:** 12

**Preparation Time:** 2 hours

**Per Serving:** Calories: 250, Protein: 24.5g, Carbs: 11.6g, Fats: 12.1g

**Ingredients:**

- 12 medium-sized bell peppers
- 2 pounds lean ground beef
- 2 onions, finely chopped
- 2 tomatoes, chopped
- 1 tsp cayenne pepper, ground
- 6 tbsps extra-virgin olive oil
- 1 tsp salt
- 1 tsp black pepper, ground

**Procedure:**

1. First, cut the stem end of each pepper and remove the seeds.
2. Rinse and set aside.

3. In a large bowl, combine ground beef, onion, tomato, cayenne pepper, olive oil, salt, and pepper.
4. Then, use two tablespoons of the mixture to fill each bell pepper.
5. Now, gently place in a large Ziploc bag and cook en sous vide for 2 hours at 140 degrees F.
6. Finally, remove the peppers from the bag and chill for about 30 minutes before serving.

# Enticing Herb Crusted Lamb Rack

**Servings:** 12

**Preparation Time:** 2 hours

**Per Serving:** Calories: 250, Protein: 14g, Carbs: 4g, Fats: 20g

**Ingredients:**

- Lamb Rack:
- 6 large Racks of Lamb
- Salt to taste
- 6 tsps Black Pepper Powder
- 2 sprig Rosemary
- 4 tbsps Olive Oil
- Herb Crust:
- 4 tbsps Fresh Rosemary Leaves
- 1 cup Macadamia Nuts
- 4 tbsps Dijon Mustard
- 1 cup Fresh Parsley
- 4 tbsps Fresh Thyme Leaves
- 4 tbsps Lemon Zest
- 4 cloves Garlic
- 4 Egg Whites

**Procedure:**

1. First, make a water bath, place the Sous Vide Cooker in it, and set to 140 degrees F.
2. Pat dry the lamb with a napkin and rub the meat with salt and black pepper.
3. Then, place a pan over medium heat and add olive oil. Sear the lamb on both sides for 8 minutes.
4. Remove and set aside.
5. Add garlic and rosemary to the pan, toast for 1 minute and pour over the lamb
6. . Remove the lamb to a plate and leave cool for 5 minutes.
7. Now, lace lamb, garlic, and rosemary in a vacuum-sealable bag, release air by the water displacement method and seal the bag.
8. Submerge the bag in the water bath. Cook for 1 hour 30 minutes.
9. Once the timer has stopped, remove the bag, unseal and take out the lamb. Whisk the egg whites and place aside.
10. Blend the remaining listed herb crust ingredients using a blender and place aside.
11. Pat dry the lamb using a napkin and brush the meat with the egg whites.

12. Dip into the herb mixture and coat graciously.
13. Place the lamb racks with crust side up on a baking sheet. Bake in an oven for 15 minutes.
14. Gently slice each cutlet.
15. Finally, serve with pureed vegetables.

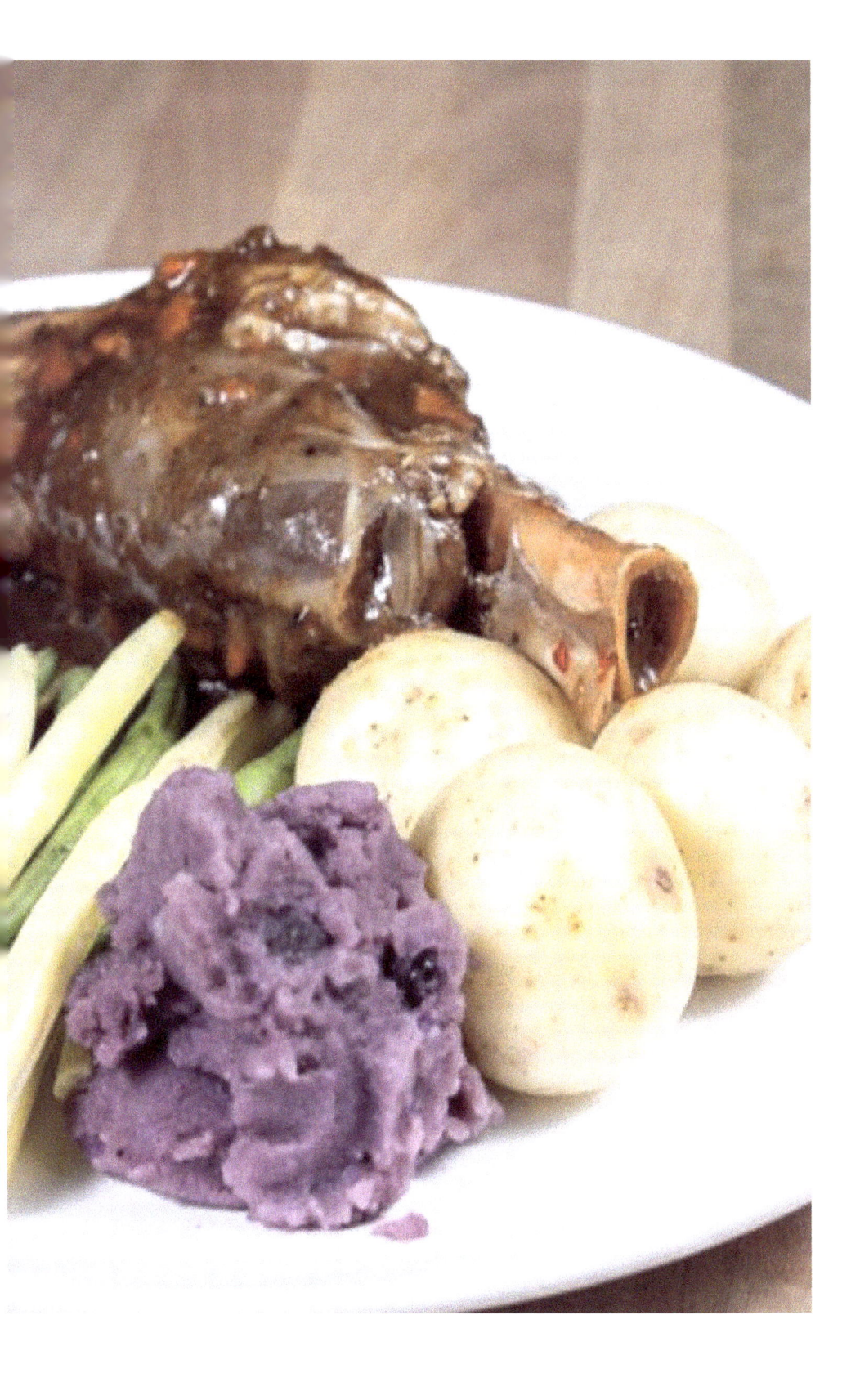

# Veal Chops

**Servings:** 8

**Preparation Time:** 3 hours

**Per Serving:** Calories: 520, Protein: 57g, Carbs: 3.4g, Fats: 17g

**Ingredients:**

- 4 (16 oz) Veal Steaks
- 4 tsps Salt
- 4 tsps Black Pepper Powder
- 4 tbsps Olive Oil

**Procedure:**

1. First, prepare a water bath, place the Sous Vide Cooker in it, and set to 135 degrees F.
2. Rub the veal with pepper and salt and place in a Ziploc bag.
3. Release air by the water displacement method and seal the bag.
4. Submerge the bag in the water bath. Cook for 3 hours. Once the timer has stopped, remove and unseal the bag.

5. Remove the veal, pat dry using a napkin, and rub with the olive oil.
6. Then, preheat a cast-iron on high heat for 5 minutes.
7. Place the steak in and sear to deeply brown on both sides.
8. Remove to a serving board.
9. Finally, serve with a side of salad.

# Enjoyable Rosemary Meatballs with Yogurt

**Servings:** 6

**Preparation Time:** 1 hour

**Per Serving:** Calories: 471 Total Fat: 24g Saturated Fat: 2g Trans Fat: 0g Protein: 43g Net Carbs: 9g Total Carbs: 8g Dietary Fiber: 8g

**Ingredients:**

- 2 pounds lean ground beef
- 6 garlic cloves, crushed
- 1/2 cup all-purpose flour
- 2 large eggs, beaten
- 2 tablespoons fresh rosemary, crushed
- 1 teaspoon sea salt
- 6 tablespoons extra-virgin olive oil
- Serve with:
- Greek yogurt and fresh parsley

**Procedure:**

1. Firstly, place the meat in a large bowl.

2. Add crushed garlic, flour, one beaten egg, fresh rosemary, salt, and oil. Combine the ingredients together.
3. Then, using your hands, shape bite-sized balls and place them in a large Ziploc.
4. Seal the bag and cook in a water bath for 1 hour at 136 degrees.
5. Now, remove from the bath and top with Greek yogurt.
6. Finally, sprinkle with some parsley and serve.

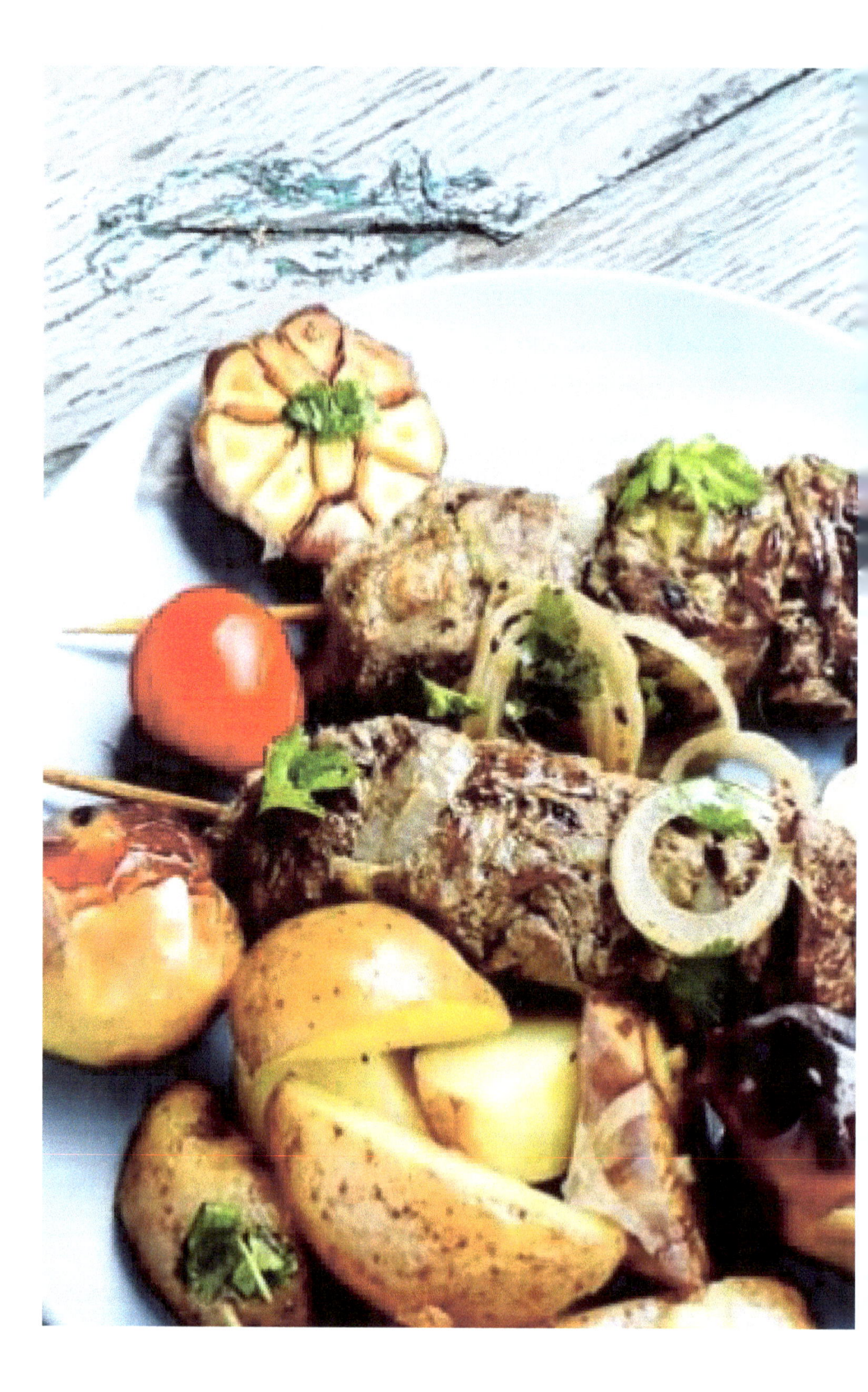

# Ground Beef Kebab

**Servings:** 8

**Preparation Time:** 1 hour

**Per Serving:** Calories: 321 Total Fat: 14g Saturated Fat: 4g Trans Fat: 0g Protein: 39g Net Carbs: 4g Total Carbs: 14g Dietary Fiber: 2g Sugars: 7g Cholesterol: 101mg Sodium: 373mg Potassium: 624mg

**Ingredients:**

- 1 pound lean ground beef
- 4 large onions, finely chopped
- 4 garlic cloves, crushed
- 4 tablespoons all-purpose flour
- 4 tablespoons vegetable oil
- 2 tablespoons tomato paste
- 2 tablespoons fresh parsley
- 1 teaspoon salt
- 1/2 teaspoon black pepper
- Serve with:
- Greek yogurt

**Procedure:**

1. First, in a large bowl, combine ground beef with onions, garlic, flour, oil, tomato paste, fresh parsley, salt, and pepper.
2. Then, mix well and shape bite-sized balls. Gently press them in the middle and transfer to a large Ziploc.
3. Now, cook en sous vide for 2 hours at 129 degrees.

# Pleasant Teriyaki Skewered Lamb

**Servings:** 4

**Preparation Time:** 3 hours

**Per Serving:** Calories: 419 Carbohydrate: 26g Protein: 39g Fat: 17g Sugar: 2g Sodium: 405mg

**Ingredients:**

- 4 lamb backstop loin steaks, cut into 2-inch cubes
- 2 tablespoons soy sauce
- 2 tablespoons mirin
- 4 tablespoons sesame oil

**Procedure:**

1. Firstly, prepare the Sous Vide water bath using your immersion circulator and raise the temperature to 140-degrees Fahrenheit
2. Add the lamb, soy and mirin in a zipper bag and seal using the immersion method
3. Cook for 3 hours

4. Now, once cooked, take the bag out from the water bath and take out the cooked lamb, pat them dry using kitchen towel
5. Thread onto skewers and discard the cooking liquid
6. Take a skillet and place it over medium-high heat, then add the oil.
7. Finally, sear both sides and serve!

# Lamb Chops & Mint Pistachio

**Servings:** 4

**Preparation Time:** 150 minutes

**Per Serving:** Calories: 474 Carbohydrate: 0g Protein: 18g Fat: 44g Sugar: 0g Sodium: 368mg

**Ingredients:**

- 2 full racks lamb sliced into chops
- Kosher salt and black pepper as needed
- 1 cup packed fresh mint leaves
- ½ cup unsalted pistachio nuts, shelled
- ½ cup packed fresh parsley
- ½ cup scallion, sliced
- 3 tablespoons lemon juice
- 2 cloves garlic, minced
- 6 tablespoons extra-virgin olive oil

**Procedure:**

1. Prepare the Sous Vide water bath using your immersion circulator and raise the temperature to 125-degrees Fahrenheit

2. Season the lamb with salt and pepper
3. Put in a zip bag and seal using the immersion method. Cook for 2 hours
4. After 20 minutes, take the lamb out and set the grill to high
5. Add the mint, parsley, pistachios, scallions, garlic, and lemon juice in a food processor and form a paste
6. Drizzle 4 tablespoons of olive oil as you process, and keep going until you have a smooth paste
7. Season with salt and pepper
8. Brush your cooked lamb with 2 tablespoons of olive oil and grill for 1 minute per side
9. Serve the chops with pesto

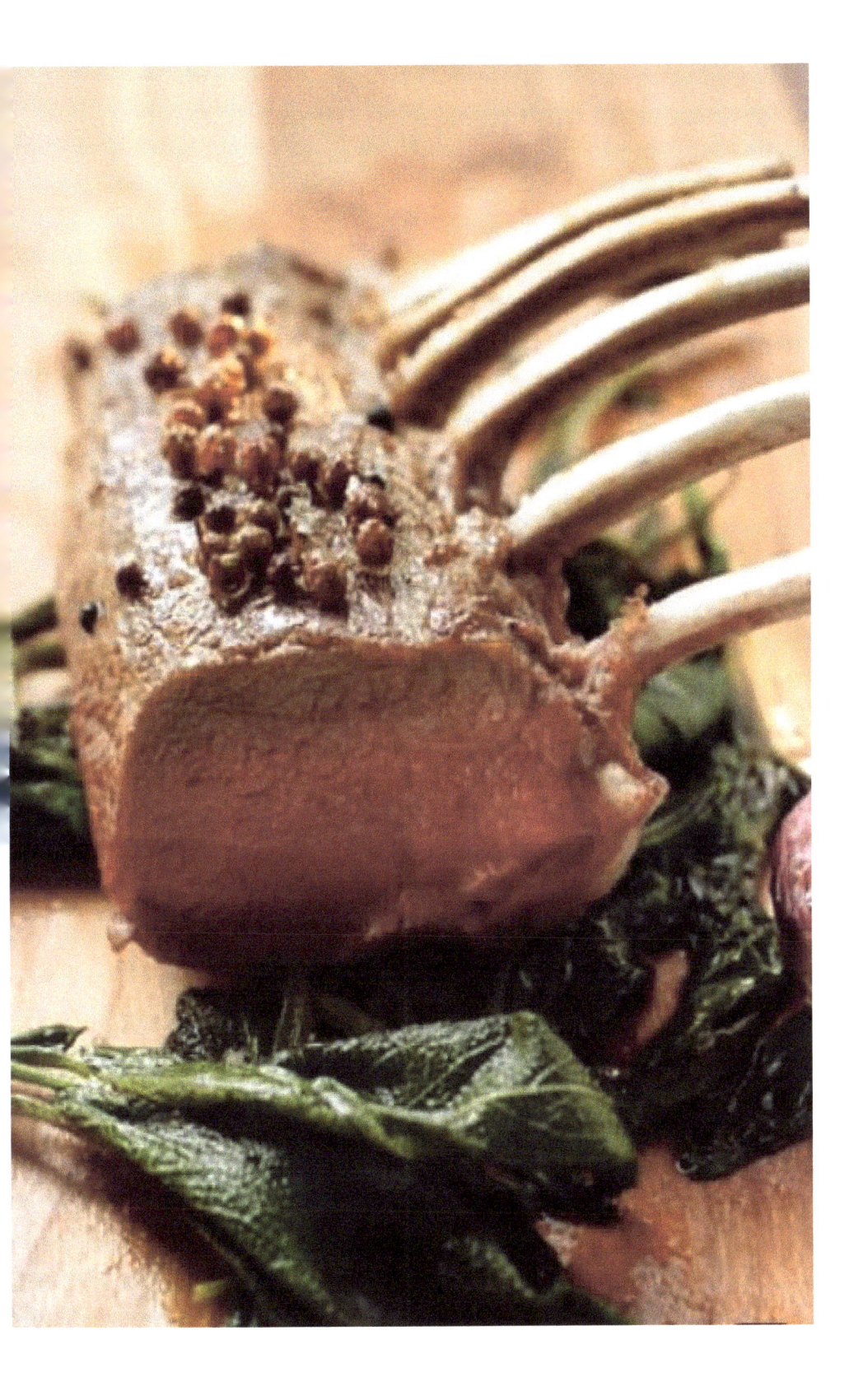

# Flavorful Lamb Rack with Dijon Mustard

**Servings:** 8

**Preparation Time:** 1 hour

**Per Serving:** Calories: 127 Carbohydrate: 5g Protein: 13g Fat: 7g Sugar: 0g Sodium: 373mg

**Ingredients:**

- 2 racks of lamb, trimmed
- 6 tablespoons honey
- 4 tablespoons Dijon mustard
- 2 teaspoons sherry vinegar
- 1/2 teaspoon salt
- 4 tablespoons avocado oil (or any oil with a high smoke point)
- Mustard seeds and chopped green onion for garnishing

**Procedure:**

1. Firstly, prepare the Sous Vide water bath using your immersion circulator and raise the temperature to 135-degrees Fahrenheit

2. Take a small-sized bowl and add all the listed ingredients (except lamb)
3. Then, mix well and place the trimmed lamb meat into a zip bag. Pour the sauce in and seal using the immersion method. Cook for 1 hour
4. Once done, take the bag out from the water bath and transfer the lamb to a serving plate; keep the juice on the side
5. Now, place a frying pan over medium-high heat, add 2 tablespoons of oil and allow it to heat up, and when it shimmers, add in the lamb and sear for 2 minutes per side
6. Slice it and drizzle the bag sauce over
7. Garnish with the mustard seeds and green onions
8. Finally, enjoy!

# Quail Breast

**Servings:** 8

**Preparation Time:** 2 hours

**Per Serving:** Calories: 320 Carbohydrate: 28g Protein: 10g Fat: 3g Sugar: 2g Sodium: 170mg

**Ingredients:**

- 16 quail breasts, bone-in, skin-on
- Kosher salt and freshly ground black pepper
- 2 tablespoons extra-virgin olive oil

**Procedure:**

1. Firstly, prepare the Sous Vide water bath using your immersion circulator and increase the temperature to 134-degrees Fahrenheit
2. Then, season the quail and place in a zip bag. Seal using the immersion method
3. Cook for 2 hours
4. Once done, remove the bag and take out the quail, pat it dry

5. Rub the cooked quail with oil
6. Now, take one cast-iron skillet and heat it. Sear the breast for 1 minute per side
7. Finally, transfer to a platter and serve

# PORK

## Pork with Tomatoes and Potatoes

**Servings:** 8

**Preparation Time:** 1 hour

**Per Serving:** Calories 253, Fat 14, Fiber 2, Carbs 6, Protein 18

**Ingredients:**

- 4 pounds pork stew meat, roughly cubed
- 2 cups cherry tomatoes, halved
- 1 pound gold potatoes, peeled and cut into wedges
- 2 teaspoons sweet paprika
- Juice of 1 lime
- 2 red onions, chopped
- 4 tablespoons avocado oil
- 6 garlic cloves, minced
- 2 tablespoons chives, chopped

**Procedure:**

1. First, in a large sous vide bag, mix the pork with the tomatoes, potatoes and the other ingredients, seal the bag, submerge in the water bath, cook at 180 degrees F for 1 hour and 40 minutes,
2. Finally, divide the mix between plates and serve.

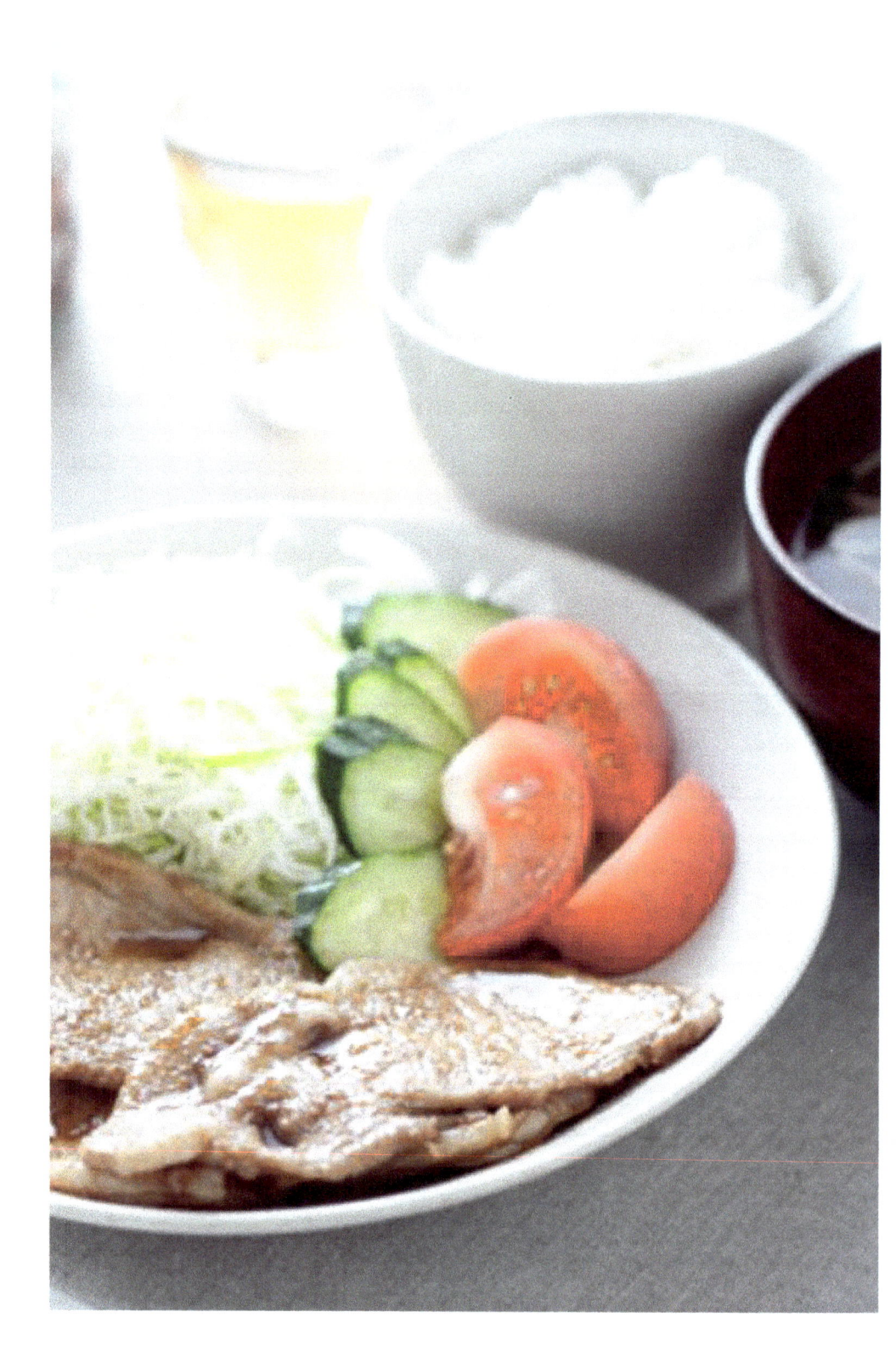

# Ginger Pork

**Servings:**

**Preparation Time:**

**Per Serving:** Calories 264, Fat 14, Fiber 2, Carbs 8, Protein 12

**Ingredients:**

- 4 pounds pork shoulder, boneless and cubed
- 4 spring onions, chopped
- 1 tablespoon ginger, grated
- 1 teaspoon chili powder
- 1 teaspoon coriander, ground
- A pinch of salt and black pepper
- ¼ cup beef stock
- 1 tablespoon cilantro, chopped

**Procedure:**

1. First, in a sous vide bag, mix the pork with the ginger, spring onions and the other ingredients, seal the bag, submerge in the water bath, cook at 175 degrees F for 1 hour and 10 minutes.
2. Finally, divide the mix between plates and serve with a side salad.

# Easy Pork and Creamy Scallions Sauce

**Servings:** 8

**Preparation Time:** 1 hour and 20 minutes

**Per Serving:** Calories 277, Fat 14, Fiber 3, Carbs 7, Protein 17

**Ingredients:**

- 4 pounds pork stew meat, cubed
- 2 cups heavy cream
- 1 cup scallions, chopped
- Juice of 1 lime
- 2 teaspoons turmeric powder
- 1 teaspoon garam masala
- 4 tablespoons olive oil
- 2 tablespoons chives, chopped
- A pinch of salt and black pepper

**Procedure:**

1. First, in a large sous vide bag, mix the pork with the cream, scallions, lime juice and the other ingredients, seal the bag, submerge in the water bath, cook at 180 degrees F for 1 hour and 20 minutes.
2. Finally, divide everything into bowls and serve.

# Delicious Pork and Zucchini Ribbons

**Servings:** 4

**Preparation Time:** 3 hours

**Per Serving:** Calories 334, Fat 33, Fiber 3, Carbs 14, Protein 7

**Ingredients:**

- 12 (6-ounce bone-in pork loin chops
- Salt and black pepper as needed
- 6 tablespoons extra-virgin olive oil
- 2 tablespoons freshly squeezed lemon juice
- 4 teaspoons red wine vinegar
- 4 teaspoons honey
- 4 tablespoons rice bran oil
- 4 medium zucchinis, sliced into ribbons
- 4 tablespoons pine nuts, toasted up

**Procedure:**

1. Firstly, prepare the Sous Vide water bath using your immersion circulator and raise the temperature to 140-degrees Fahrenheit.

2. Then, take the pork chops and season it with salt and pepper, transfer to a heavy-duty zip bag and add 1 tablespoon of oil.
3. Seal using the immersion method and cook for 3 hours.
4. Prepare the dressing by whisking lemon juice, honey, vinegar, 2 tablespoons of olive oil and season with salt and pepper.
5. Once cooked, remove the bag from the water bath and discard the liquid.
6. Heat up rice bran oil in a large skillet over high heat and add the pork chops, sear until browned (1 minute per side
7. Once done, transfer it to a cutting board and allow it to rest for 5 minutes.
8. Now, take a medium bowl and add the zucchini ribbons with dressing
9. Thinly slice the pork chops and discard the bone.
10. Place the pork on top of the zucchini.
11. Finally, top with pine nuts and serve!

# Tasty Herbed Pork Loin

**Servings:** 8

**Preparation Time:** 2 hours

**Per Serving:** Calories 334, Fat 33, Fiber 3, Carbs 14, Protein 7

**Ingredients:**

- 2 (1 lb. pork tenderloin, trimmed
- Salt and fresh ground pepper as needed
- 2 tablespoons chopped fresh basil + additional for servings
- 2 tablespoons chopped fresh parsley + additional for servings
- 2 tablespoons chopped fresh rosemary + additional for servings
- 4 tablespoons unsalted butter

**Procedure:**

1. Firstly, prepare the Sous Vide water bath using your immersion circulator and raise the temperature to 134-degrees Fahrenheit. Season the tenderloin with pepper and salt

2. Rub herbs (a mixture of basil, parsley and rosemary all over the tenderloin and transfer to a resalable zip bag
3. Add 1 tablespoon of butter
4. Seal using the immersion method. Submerge underwater and cook for 2 hours
5. Then, once cooked, remove the bag and remove the pork from the bag
6. Place a large-sized skillet over medium-high heat
7. Add the remaining butter and herb mixture and allow the butter to heat up
8. Add the pork and sear it well for 1-2 minutes on each side, making sure to keep scooping the butter over the pork
9. Now, remove the heat and transfer the pork to a cutting board
10. Allow it to rest for 5 minutes and slice into medallions
11. Finally, serve with extra herbs and a sprinkle of salt

# Enjoyable Red Pepper Salad and Pork Chops

**Servings:** 8

**Preparation Time:** 1 hour

**Per Serving:** Calories 334, Fat 33, Fiber 3, Carbs 14, Protein 7

**Ingredients:**

- 4 pork chops
- 2 small red bell peppers, diced
- 2 small yellow onions, diced
- 4 cups frozen corn kernels
- 1/2 cup cilantro, chopped
- Salt and pepper as needed
- Vegetable oil as needed

**Procedure:**

1. First, prepare the Sous Vide water bath using your immersion circulator and raise the temperature to 140-degrees Fahrenheit.
2. Season the pork carefully with salt
3. Then, transfer the pork to a resealable zip bag and seal using the immersion method.

4. Submerge underwater and cook for 1 hour
5. Take a pan and put it over medium heat and add the oil; allow it to heat up
6. Add the onion, red pepper, corn and sauté for a while until they are slightly browned
7. Season with salt and pepper
8. Finish the corn mix with a garnish of chopped cilantro, keep it aside
9. Remove the pan from heat and wipe the oil
10. Place it back to medium-high heat
11. Put the oil and allow it to heat up
12. Now, transfer the cooked pork chops to the pan and sear each side for 1 minute
13. Finally, serve the pork chops with the salad!

# Pleasant Fragrant Nonya Pork Belly

**Servings:** 4

**Preparation Time:** 7 hours

**Per Serving:** Calories 334, Fat 33, Fiber 3, Carbs 14, Protein 7

**Ingredients:**

- 1/2 lb. pork belly
- 1.8 cup chopped shallots
- 3 sliced garlic cloves
- 1/4 tablespoon coriander seeds
- 1-star anise
- 2 large dried shiitake mushrooms
- 1 tablespoon coconut aminos
- 1 teaspoon brown sugar
- 1/2 teaspoon salt
- 1/8 teaspoon ground white pepper

**Procedure:**

1. Firstly, prepare the Sous Vide water bath using your immersion circulator and raise the temperature to 176-degrees Fahrenheit.

2. Chop up the pork belly into 1-inch cubes and transfer to a bowl.
3. Add the remaining ingredients and whisk them well.
4. Transfer to a resealable zip bag and seal using the immersion method.
5. Then, cook for 7 hours and remove the bag.
6. Transfer the solids to servings dish and discard the star anise.
7. Now, tip the cooking liquid to a small pan and reduce it over medium heat.
8. Now, pour the sauce over pork belly and serve!

# Enjoyable Pork Chop with Corn

**Servings:** 6

**Preparation Time:** 1 hour

**Per Serving:** Calories: 353 Carbohydrate: 8g Protein: 41g Fat: 16g Sugar: 4g Sodium: 162mg

**Ingredients:**

- 8 pieces pork chop
- 2 small red bell peppers, diced
- 2 small yellow onions, diced
- 6 ears corn kernels
- 1/2 cup cilantro, chopped
- Salt and pepper as needed
- Vegetable oil

**Procedure:**

1. Firstly, prepare the Sous Vide water bath using your immersion circulator and raise the temperature to 140-degrees Fahrenheit.
2. Season the pork chop with salt.

3. Then, transfer to a resealable zip bag and seal using the immersion method. Cook for 1 hour.
4. Take a pan and put it over medium heat, add the oil and allow the oil to heat up
5. Add the onion, corn, and bell pepper.
6. Sauté for a while until barely browned.
7. Now, finish the corn mix with cilantro and set it aside.
8. Wipe the pan clean and place the pan over medium heat.
9. Add the oil and sear the pork chop for 1 minute per side.
10. Finally, slice and serve with the salad.

# Mango Salsa and Pork

**Servings:** 8

**Preparation Time:** 2 hours

**Per Serving:** Calories: 217 Carbohydrate: 11g Protein: 25g Fat: 8g Sugar: 8g Sodium: 112mg

**Ingredients:**

- 1/2 cup light broth sugar
- 2 tablespoons ground allspice
- 1 teaspoon cayenne pepper
- 1/2 teaspoon ground cinnamon
- 1/2 teaspoon ground cloves
- Kosher salt and black pepper, as needed
- 4 lbs pork tenderloin
- 4 tablespoons canola oil
- 4 pitted and peeled mangoes, finely diced
- 1/2 cup fresh cilantro, chopped
- 2 red bell pepper, stemmed, seeded, and finely diced
- 6 tablespoons red onion, finely diced
- 4 tablespoons freshly squeezed lime juice
- 2 small jalapenos seeded and finely diced

**Procedure:**

1. Firstly, prepare the Sous Vide water bath using your immersion circulator and raise the temperature to 135-degrees Fahrenheit.
2. Then, take a medium bowl and mix the sugar, allspice, cinnamon, cayenne, cloves, 2 teaspoons of salt, and 1 teaspoon of pepper.
3. Rub the mixture over the tenderloins.
4. Take a large-sized skillet and put it over medium heat, add the oil and once the oil simmers, transfer the pork and sear for 5 minutes, browning all sides.
5. Transfer to a plate and rest for 10 minutes.
6. Transfer the pork chop to a resealable zipper bag and seal using the immersion method. Cook for 2 hours.
7. Once cooked, take the bag out and allow it to rest for a while, take the chop out and slice it.
8. Now, prepare the salsa by mixing the mango, cilantro, bell pepper, onion, lime juice, and jalapeno in a mixing bowl.
9. Finally, serve the sliced pork with salsa with a seasoning salt and pepper.

# Tempting Lemongrass Pork Chops

**Servings:** 4

**Preparation Time:** 2 hours

**Per Serving:** Calories: 262 Carbohydrate: 12g Protein: 26g Fat: 12g Sugar: 1.2g Sodium: 458mg

**Ingredients:**

- 4 tablespoons coconut oil
- 2 stalks sliced lemon grass
- 2 tablespoons minced shallot
- 2 tablespoons soy sauce
- 2 tablespoons mirin
- 2 tablespoons rice wine vinegar
- 2 tablespoons light brown sugar
- 2 teaspoons minced fresh ginger
- 2 teaspoons fish sauce
- 2 teaspoons kosher salt
- 4 (10-ounce) bone-in pork rib chops
- 2 teaspoons minced garlic

**Procedure:**

1. First, prepare the Sous Vide water bath using your immersion circulator and raise the temperature to 140-degrees Fahrenheit.
2. Take a food processor and add 1 tablespoon of coconut oil, lemon grass, soy sauce, shallot, vinegar, mirin, brown sugar, garlic, fish sauce, ginger, and salt.
3. Process for 1 minute.
4. Then, place the pork chops into a resealable zip bag alongside soy-lemon grass mixture and seal using the immersion method. Cook for 2 hours.
5. Once cooked, remove the bag and take the pork chops out, pat them dry.
6. Heat a grill to high heat and sear the chops until well browned.
7. Now, allow it to rest for 2-3 minutes.
8. Finally, serve!

# Enticing Pork and Zucchini Ribbons

**Servings:** 4

**Preparation Time:** 3 hours

**Per Serving:** Calories: 174 Carbohydrate: 4g Protein: 19g Fat: 9g Sugar: 2g Sodium: 302mg

**Ingredients:**

- 4 (6-ounce) bone-in pork loin chops
- Salt and black pepper as needed
- 6 tablespoons extra-virgin olive oil
- 2 tablespoons freshly squeezed lemon juice
- 4 teaspoons red wine vinegar
- 4 teaspoons honey
- 4 tablespoons rice bran oil
- 4 medium zucchini, sliced into ribbons
- 4 tablespoons pine nuts, toasted up

**Procedure:**

1. First, prepare the Sous Vide water bath using your immersion circulator and raise the temperature to 140-degrees Fahrenheit.

2. Take the pork chops and season it with salt and pepper, transfer to a heavy-duty zip bag and add 1 tablespoon of oil.
3. Seal using the immersion method and cook for 3 hours.
4. Prepare the dressing by whisking lemon juice, honey, vinegar, 2 tablespoons of olive oil and season with salt and pepper.
5. Then, once cooked, remove the bag from the water bath and discard the liquid.
6. Heat up rice bran oil in a large skillet over high heat and add the pork chops, sear until browned (1 minute per side)
7. Once done, transfer it to a cutting board and allow to rest for 5 minutes.
8. Take a medium bowl and add the zucchini ribbons with dressing
9. Thinly slice the pork chops and discard the bone.
10. Now, place the pork on top of the zucchini.
11. Finally, top with pine nuts and serve!

# Easy Herbed Pork Loin

**Servings:** 8

**Preparation Time:** 2 hours

**Per Serving:** Calories: 284 Carbohydrate: 3g Protein: 33g Fat: 14g Sugar: 0g Sodium: 421mg

**Ingredients:**

- 2 (1 lb.) pork tenderloin, trimmed
- Salt and fresh ground pepper as needed
- 2 tablespoons chopped fresh basil + additional for serving
- 2 tablespoons chopped fresh parsley + additional for serving
- 2 tablespoons chopped fresh rosemary + additional for serving
- 4 tablespoons unsalted butter

**Procedure:**

1. Firstly, prepare the Sous Vide water bath using your immersion circulator and raise the temperature to 134-

degrees Fahrenheit. Season the tenderloin with pepper and salt
2. Rub herbs (a mixture of basil, parsley and rosemary) all over the tenderloin and transfer to a resalable zip bag
3. Add 1 tablespoon of butter
4. Seal using the immersion method. Submerge underwater and cook for 2 hours
5. Once cooked, remove the bag and remove the pork from the bag
6. Place a large-sized skillet over medium–high heat
7. Now, add the remaining butter and herb mixture and allow the butter to heat up
8. Add the pork and sear it well for 1-2 minutes each side, making sure to keep scooping the butter over the pork
9. Remove the heat and transfer the pork to a cutting board
10. Allow it to rest for 5 minutes and slice into medallions
11. Finally, serve with extra herbs and a sprinkle of salt

# SIDE DISHES

# Tasty Trout with Pesto and Lemon Juice

**Servings:** 4

**Preparation Time:** 40 minute

**Per Serving:** Calories: 352 Protein: 35 g Fats: 22 g Carbs: 1 g

**Ingredients:**

- 4 medium fish fillets of your choice (salmon, cod, trout or other)
- 4 tbsps olive oil
- Salt and pepper to taste
- 8 tbsps Pesto sauce
- 4 tbsps lemon juice

**Procedure:**

1. Firstly, preheat the water bath to 135 degrees F.
2. Rub the trout fillets with salt, pepper and pesto sauce, and put the fish and olive oil into the vacuum bag.
3. Then, seal the bag and set the timer for 30 minutes.
4. Finally, serve sprinkled with lemon juice.

# Easy Garlic and Herbs Cod

**Servings:** 4

**Preparation Time:** 40 minutes

**Per Serving:** Calories: 250 Protein: 22 g Fats: 8 g Carbs: 18 g

**Ingredients:**

- 4 medium cod fillets
- 4 garlic cloves, minced
- 2 tbsps fresh rosemary, chopped
- 2 tbsps fresh thyme, chopped
- 4 tbsps unsalted butter
- 2 tbsps olive oil
- Juice of 1 lemon
- Salt and pepper to taste

**Procedure:**

1. Firstly, preheat the water bath to 135 degrees F.
2. Then, rub the cod fillets with salt and pepper, and put them into the vacuum bag, adding rosemary, thyme, butter, minced garlic and lemon juice.
3. Now, seal the bag and set the timer for 30 minutes.
4. When the time is up, sear the fish in a cast-iron skillet in 1 tbsp olive oil on both sides and serve over white rice.

# Delicious Coconut Cream Sea Bass

**Servings:** 4

**Preparation Time:** 40 minutes

**Per Serving:** Calories: 580 Protein: 22 g Fats: 15 g Carbs: 88 g

**Ingredients:**

For the fish

- 4 medium cod fillets
- 4 tbsps coconut milk
- Salt and pepper to taste

For the sauce

- 1 cup coconut milk
- 1 cup chicken broth
- 1 tsp white sugar
- 2 tsps lime juice
- 4 slices ginger root
- Chopped cilantro for serving

**Procedure:**

1. Firstly, preheat the water bath to 135 degrees F.
2. Rub the sea bass fillets with salt, pepper, and coconut milk and put them into the vacuum bag.
3. Then, seal the bag and set the timer for 30 minutes.
4. While the fish is cooking, make the sauce.
5. Combine the chicken broth and coconut milk in a pan, and simmer for about 10 minutes over medium heat.
6. Add the lime juice, sugar and ginger root, mix well and take the sauce off the heat.
7. Now, close the pan with the lid and set aside for a couple of minutes.
8. Finally, put the fish in bowls, pour the sauce over and serve topped with the freshly chopped cilantro.

# Wild Salmon Steaks

**Servings:** 8

**Preparation Time:** 55 minutes

**Per Serving:** Calories: 324, Protein: 39.7g, Carbs: 29.3g, Fats: 5.2g

**Ingredients:**

- 4 pounds wild salmon steaks
- 6 garlic cloves, crushed
- 2 tbsps fresh rosemary, chopped
- 2 tbsps lemon juice
- 2 tbsps orange juice
- 2 tsps orange zest
- 2 tsps pink Himalayan salt
- 2 cups fish stock

**Procedure:**

1. Firstly, combine orange juice with lemon juice, rosemary, garlic, orange zest, and salt.
2. Brush the mixture over each steak and refrigerate for 20 minutes.

3. Then, transfer to a Ziploc bag and add fish stock. Seal the bag and cook en sous vide for 45 minutes at 131 degrees F.
4. Preheat a large, non-stick grill pan.
5. Now, remove the steaks from Ziploc and grill for 3 minutes on each side, until lightly charred.

# Enticing Marinated Catfish Fillets

**Servings:** 6

**Preparation Time:** 1 hour

**Per Serving:** Calories: 368, Protein: 25.1g, Carbs: 8.7g, Fats: 26.3g

**Ingredients:**

- 2 pounds catfish fillet
- 1 cup lemon juice
- 1 cup parsley, chopped
- 4 garlic cloves, crushed
- 2 cups onions, finely chopped
- 2 tbsps fresh dill, chopped
- 2 tbsps rosemary, chopped
- 4 cups apple juice
- 4 tbsps Dijon mustard
- 2 cups extra virgin olive oil

**Procedure:**

1. First, in a large bowl, combine lemon juice, parsley leaves, crushed garlic, finely chopped onions, fresh dill, rosemary, apple juice, mustard, and olive oil.
2. Whisk together until well incorporated.

3. Submerge fillets in this mixture and cover with a tight lid. Refrigerate for 30 minutes.
4. Remove from the refrigerator and place in 2 separate Ziploc bags.
5. Then, seal the bags, and cook en sous vide for 40 minutes at 129 degrees F.
6. Now, remove from the bags and drain but make sure to reserve the liquid.
7. Finally, transfer to a serving platter and drizzle with its liquid.

# Enjoyable Cilantro Trout

**Servings:** 8

**Preparation Time:** 1 hour

**Per Serving:** Calories: 567, Protein: 57.9g, Carbs: 2.8g, Fats: 33.6g

**Ingredients:**

- 4 pounds trout, 4 pieces
- 10 garlic cloves
- 2 tbsps sea salt
- 8 tbsps olive oil
- 2 cups cilantro leaves, chopped
- 4 tbsps rosemary, chopped
- 1/2 cup lemon juice

**Procedure:**

1. Firstly, rub the fish with salt.
2. Combine garlic with olive oil, cilantro, rosemary, and lemon juice. Use the mixture to fill each fish.
3. Then, place in a Ziploc bag and seal.
4. Now, cook en sous vide for 55 minutes at 120 degrees F.

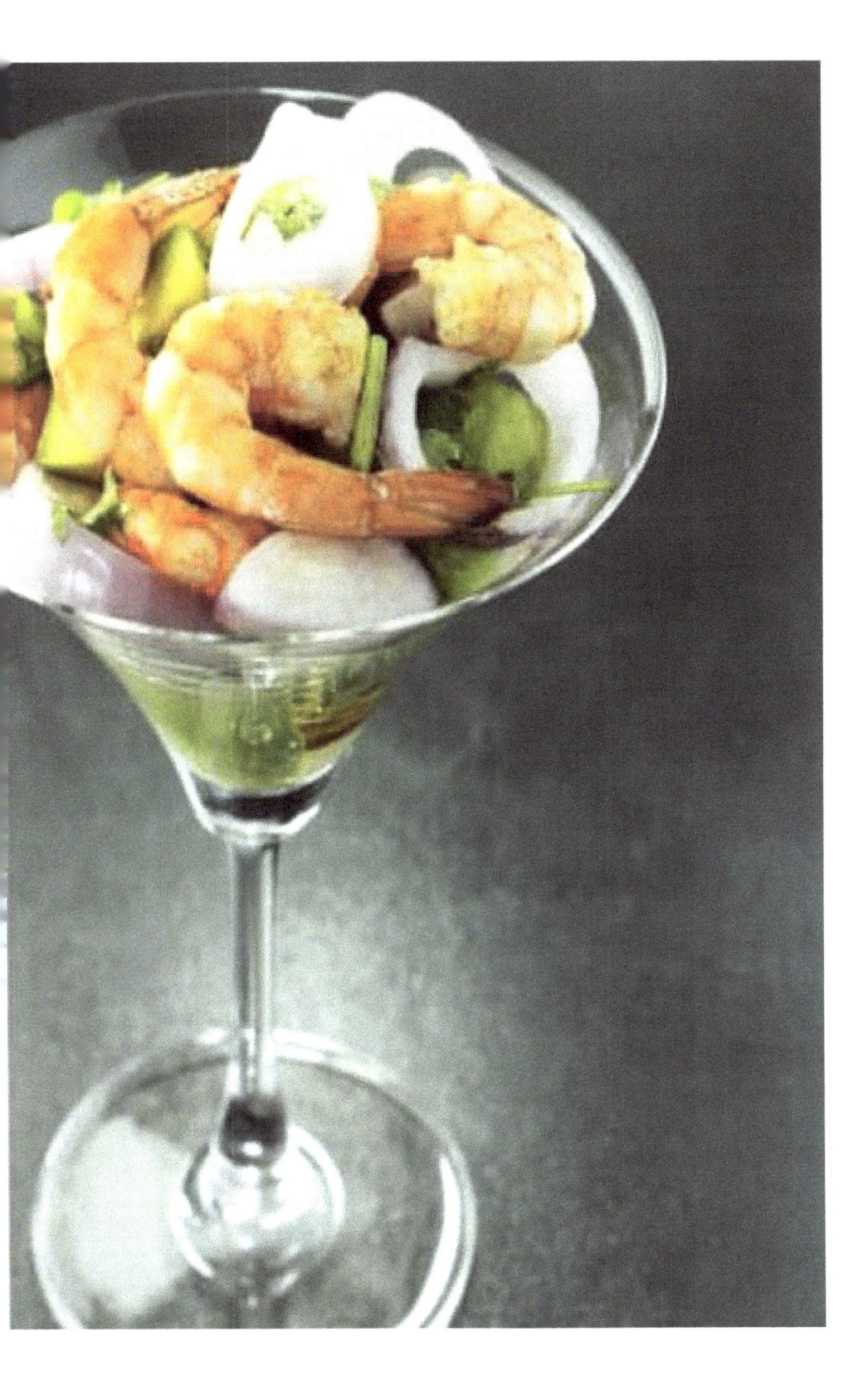

# Shrimp Salad

**Servings:** 8

**Preparation Time:** 40 minutes

**Per Serving:** Calories 142, Carbohydrates 7 g, Fats 2 g, Protein 24 g

**Ingredients:**

- 2 chopped red onions
- Juice, 2 limes
- 2 teaspoons extra-virgin olive oil
- 1/2 teaspoon sea salt
- 1/2 teaspoon white pepper
- 2 lbs raw shrimp, peeled, deveined
- 2 diced tomatoes
- 2 diced avocados
- 2 jalapenos, seeded, diced
- 2 tablespoons chopped cilantro

**Procedure:**

1. Firstly, prepare your Sous-vide water bath to a temperature of 148ºF

2. Add the lime juice, red onion, sea salt, white pepper, extra virgin olive oil, white pepper and shrimp into your heavy-duty plastic bag
3. Then, seal the bag using the immersion method
4. Submerge the bag underwater and cook for 24 minutes
5. Remove and chill the plastic bag in an ice bath for about 10 minutes
6. Now, take a large-sized bowl and add the tomato, avocado, jalapeno and cilantro
7. Remove it from the bag and top it up with the salad.
8. Finally, serve!

# Shrimp and Leek

**Servings:** 8

**Preparation Time:** 1 hour

**Per Serving:** Calories: 148 Carbohydrate: 7g Protein: 24g Fat: 2g Sugar: 3g Sodium: 758mg

**Ingredients:**

- 12 leeks
- 10 tablespoons extra-virgin olive oil
- Kosher salt as needed
- Freshly ground black pepper
- 2 small-sized shallots, minced
- 2 tablespoons champagne vinegar
- 2 teaspoons Dijon mustard
- 1 lb cooked bay shrimp
- Chopped fresh parsley for garnishing

**Procedure:**

1. Firstly, prepare your Sous-vide water bath to a temperature of 183-degrees Fahrenheit
2. Cut off the top of your leeks and discard them

3. Trim the root ends of each leek and wash them in cold water
4. Brush the leek with 1 tablespoon of olive oil
5. Then, season with salt and put the leeks in a large-sized zipper bag and seal it using the immersion method
6. Submerge the bag underwater and cook for about 1 hour
7. To make the vinaigrette, take a small-sized bowl and whisk the shallot, Dijon mustard, vinegar and ¼ cup of olive oil all together. Season with some salt and pepper.
8. Once cooked, remove the bag from the water bath and transfer it to an ice bath. Chill the leeks
9. Now, divide the leeks between four plates and season them with salt
10. Top the leeks with the bay shrimp and spoon on some vinaigrette
11. Finally, sprinkle with fresh parsley and serve!

# Tasty Pumpkin Shrimp

**Servings:** 12

**Preparation Time:** 40 minutes

**Per Serving:** Calories: 221 Carbohydrate: 11g Protein: 17g Fat: 14g Sugar: 3g Sodium: 852mg

**Ingredients:**

- 16 large raw shrimps, peeled and deveined
- 1 tablespoon butter
- Salt and pepper as needed
- For Soup
- 2 lbs pumpkin
- 8 tablespoons lime juice
- 4 yellow onions, chopped
- 4 small red chilies, finely chopped
- 2 stem of lemon grass, white part only, chopped
- 2 teaspoons shrimp paste
- 2 teaspoons sugar
- 3 cups coconut milk
- 2 teaspoons tamarind paste
- 2 cups water

- 1 cup coconut cream
- 2 tablespoons fish sauce
- 4 tablespoons fresh Thai basil, chopped

**Procedure:**

1. Firstly, prepare your Sous-vide water bath to a temperature of 122-degrees Fahrenheit
2. Add the shrimps into your Sous Vide bag with the butter
3. Sprinkle salt and pepper in and seal the bag using the immersion method and cook for 15-35 minutes
4. Then, peel the pumpkin and remove the seeds. Cut the flesh into 1-inch chunks
5. Add the onion, lemon grass, chili, shrimp paste, sugar and ½ the coconut milk into a food processor. Mix them well
6. Add the onion puree, remaining coconut milk, tamarind paste and water into a separate pot
7. Now, put the pumpkin to this pot and bring to a boil
8. Once the boiling point is reached, lower down the heat and simmer for 10 minutes
9. Remove the shrimps from the bag and add them to the soup

10. Add in the coconut cream, fish sauce, lime juice and basil, stir them well.
11. Finally, serve!

**Special Tips**

- You may roast the pumpkin seeds in canola oil (at 300-degrees Fahrenheit) in an oven for about 10-20 minutes and use them as garnish for an extra flavor.

# Enjoyable Miso Butter Cod

**Servings:** 4

**Preparation Time:** 40 minutes

**Per Serving:** Calories: 309 Carbohydrate: 7g Protein: 38g Fat: 15g Sugar: 1g Sodium: 806mg

**Ingredients:**

- 2 large Atlantic Cod fillet
- 4 tablespoons miso paste
- 3 tablespoons brown sugar
- 4 tablespoons soy sauce
- 4 tablespoons mirin
- 4 tablespoons butter
- Sesame seeds for garnishing

**Procedure:**

1. First, prepare your Sous-vide water bath to a temperature of 131-degrees Fahrenheit
2. Marinate the cod with the brown sugar, miso paste, mirin and soy sauce mixture

3. Transfer the fish to a heavy-duty sous vide zip bag and seal it using the immersion method
4. Cook for 30 minutes
5. Place a pan over medium heat. Add in 1 tablespoon of butter
6. Sear the cod for 1 minute and pour the juices from the bag into the pan
7. Now, reduce until it thickened and add 1 tablespoon of butter on top and stir
8. Drizzle the sauce onto the cod and garnish with some sesame seeds
9. Finally, serve over steamed rice!

# Yummy Dijon Cream Sauce with Salmon

**Servings:** 4

**Preparation Time:** 1 hour

**Per Serving:** Calories: 204 Carbohydrate: 7g Protein: 28g Fat: 8g Sugar: 3g Sodium: 489mg

**Ingredients:**

- 8 skinless salmon fillets
- 2 bunches of spinach
- 1 cup Dijon mustard
- 2 cups heavy cream
- 2 tablespoons lemon juice
- Salt and pepper as needed

**Procedure:**

1. Firstly, prepare your Sous-vide water bath to a temperature of 115-degrees Fahrenheit
2. Season the salmon with salt
3. Transfer to a resealable bag and seal using the immersion method. Cook for 45 minutes

4. Then, take a pan and place it on medium heat and add the spinach and cook until wilted
5. Add the lemon juice, pepper and salt, and keep cooking over a low heat
6. Take another saucepan and place it over medium heat
7. Add the heavy cream and Dijon mustard. Let it all boil a bit and then lower down the heat.
8. Now, mix them well and season with salt and pepper
9. Finally, take out the cooked salmon, drizzle the sauce on top, assemble the spinach on the side, and serve!

# Flavorful Mahi-Mahi Corn Salad

**Servings:** 8

**Preparation Time:** 40 minutes

**Per Serving:** Calories: 412 Carbohydrate: 24g Protein: 44g Fat: 6g Sugar: 18g Sodium: 385mg

**Ingredients:**

- 8 mahi-mahi portions
- 1 teaspoon paprika
- 1 teaspoon onion powder
- 1 teaspoon garlic powder
- 1/2 teaspoon cayenne pepper
- Salt and pepper as needed

For the Salad

- 6 cups corn
- 1 pint cherry tomatoes, halved
- 2 red bell peppers, diced
- 4 tablespoons fresh basil, chopped

For dressing

- 4 tablespoons lime juice
- 2 teaspoons ancho chile powder
- 2 tablespoons olive oil
- Salt and pepper as needed

For garnishing

- Lime wedge
- 2 tablespoons fresh basil

**Procedure:**

1. Firstly, prepare your Sous-vide water bath to a temperature of 122-degrees Fahrenheit
2. Season the mahi-mahi fillet with salt and pepper and put it in a sous vide zip bag.
3. Then, whisk together the garlic powder, paprika, onion powder, and cayenne.
4. Sprinkle the spice mix on top of the fish and seal the bag.
5. Transfer the bag to the water bath and cook for 15-35 minutes
6. Now, preheat the oven to 400-degrees Fahrenheit
7. Add the corn and red pepper on a baking tray.

8. Drizzle the olive oil over the top with salt and pepper.
9. Cook until the corn kernels are soft.
10. In a bowl, mix the cooked corn, roasted red peppers, tomatoes, and basil and whisk them well. In another bowl mix well the ingredients for the dressing and pour over the corn kernels.
11. Take the Mahi-mahi fillet out of the bag and pat dry.
12. Sear over high-heat in a pan about 2 minutes per side.
13. For serving, take a large spoonful of the corn mix and place on the plates.
14. Finally, add the mahi-mahi fillet on top. Garnish with lime wedge and basil. Serve!

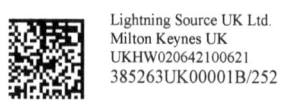

Lightning Source UK Ltd.
Milton Keynes UK
UKHW020642100621
385263UK00001B/252